Endorsements

As both a healthcare provider and empowered patient who practiced a Ketogenic lifestyle while healing from a rare spinal cord injury, Dr. Sharnael Wolverton Sehon hit a homerun with her latest book living the Ketogenic lifestyle. With her warm writing style infused in every chapter, reading this book was like having a conversation with a good friend.

In an easy to understand manner, this book will empower any reader physically, emotionally, and spiritually. Dr. Wolverton Sehon strategically guides you through 31 days of education and practical application of the Keto lifestyle. As with any lifestyle change, it can be easy to become overwhelmed and want to give up. Dr. Wolverton Sehon touches on many of the speed bumps that are encountered when first starting Ketogenic eating, offering solutions and easy to implement tips for everyday life. Day 17: Starbucks Hacks will be a delicious lifesaver!

The incorporation of additional resources and an introduction to other important topics critical to healing – such as sleep, mindset, crystals, and essential oils – provide the reader with an overall strategy for beginning their journey to optimal health and finding success. I highly recommend *Keto Reset* as a fantastic ground zero resource for my patients looking to empower themselves through a Ketogenic lifestyle.

Dr. Nevada Gray, PharmD, RN
The PALEO Pharmacist
ThePaleoPharmacist.com

As a pharmacist and author of the *Clean Slate Cleanse*, I love seeing health and wellness practitioners take an interest in diet. Dr. Wolverton Sehon is a naturopath who brings her passion for Keto to life in *Keto Reset*. She makes the transition easy and backs it with scientific research.

Lindsey Elmore, PharmD, BCPS
Author of *Essentials: 50 Answers to Common Questions about Essential Oils* and *Clean Slate Cleanse Cookbook and Workbook*
LindseyElmore.com

Dr. Sharnael is a wealth of knowledge and a great teacher on all things related to health and wellness. In this book she has done a fantastic job describing not only the benefits of a Keto lifestyle but practical examples of how to accomplish it. A great read that is both simple and useful.

Dr. Jim Bob Haggerton
DoctorJimBob.com
OilyApp.com

Keto Reset with Dr. Sharnael is a must have in your health and wellness library. She teaches simple daily steps on how to feel and look your best. Unlike other programs on the market, Dr. Sharnael encourages, supports, and problem solves for most all ages, body types, and challenges.

My own personal results were phenomenal. Forty-eight hours into the program, I was feeling the best I had in years. By day five my cravings were gone and I could easily say no to my "favorite sweets." At twelve days my mental clarity and productivity were at an all time high. By the end of the reset, my body looked amazing and my mind felt amazing.

If you are serious about improving your health, having more energy, incredible mental clarity, and the body of your dreams, you need this book!

Dr. Mary Starr Carter
The Total Wellness Doc and Mom
TheTotalWellnessDoc.com

Dr. Sharnael Wolverton Sehon has written a must-read educational guide full of valuable information for those wanting to enjoy the health benefits of a Keto lifestyle, including the importance of intermittent fasting, exercise, and reading product labels (my favorite!). Read this book and learn from one of the best.

Stacey Kimbrell
Author of *Living Balanced Reference Guide*
LivingAnointed.com

The *Keto Reset* is a must read for anyone who is looking to reclaim their health. The time is now! Dr. Sharnael Wolverton Sehon provides you with this amazing resource, which is a culmination of her own healing journey and years of experience helping others successfully implement the Keto lifestyle. This easy-to-follow program will help you finally lose the weight and feel so much better! I highly recommend you grab a copy of this book. The tools and information will provide you with an easy-to-follow, step-by-step guide that will transform your health.

Dr. Pia Martin DC, CCN, CWC, CHC
Best Selling Author of *Building Healthy Humans*
DrPia.com

Dr. Sharnael again, eloquently explains in the *Keto Reset* the journey of a Keto life. She lives this life, so she understands the pitfalls along the way. She shares from the heart how to best live the Keto lifestyle, and shares tips of biohacking the metabolism for a more efficient metabolism. She makes what appears to be difficult, simple, so others can live this life too. I highly endorse Dr. Sharnael and this book.

Thomas Lucky MD, P(MD)
Unleashing the Healing Miracle Within
TheFlowClinic.com

Keto Reset
31 Days to New Life

Dr. Sharnael Wolverton Sehon

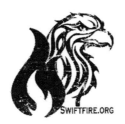

SWIFTFIRE.ORG

For more information about our products or services, please visit our website or contact:
www.swiftfire.org or www.drsharnael.com
Dr. Sharnael Wolverton Sehon
sharnael@swiftfire.org

Swiftfire Publishing

Publishers Cataloging-in-Publication Data
Keto Reset.; by Sharnael Wolverton Sehon
136 pages cm.
ISBN: 9780979662232 paperback
        9780979662249 eBook
        9780979662256 eBook
Printed in the United States of America

Dedication

I have several amazing people I am so forever thankful to:
My Creator for giving me the dreams and instruction to quit sugar to stay on the planet, my parents Chris and Connie, my Divine Love - Brian - and my beautiful kiddos Shaen and Austin, Søren, Ava, Sharnael, and Adam.

I am thankful for Dr. Gary Young, Doug Addison, Dr. Thomas Lucky, and Robert Tennyson Stevens for helping me RE-Member my divine health!

To my Keto peeps in our 31 Days to Life Keto Reset membership group—OMG! you inspire me every day!

Thank you, thank you!

Also special love to Colleen Higgs, Christal Washington, Olivia Bennett, Renee Jones, Jessica Barnett, Sarah Blair, Jeanni and Don Ellis, Alma Walker, Gene and Terri Backlund, Teresa Wages, Tanya Jaufre, Lisa McCorkle, Karlyn Abdalla, Candace Guidry, Caroline Boudreau, and Anna Fogg.

You all are my inspiration and you inspire so many! Keep being Light!

You ALL mean more than any words could ever say.

To everyone who has followed and supported me over the years on this journey—whether on social media, in my classes, at conferences, etc.—over, in, and through all our transformation together, all through the years...You are my people and I adore you.

Thanks to Marti Statler, Kevin Lepp (cover), and Shannon Johnson (editor).

Table of Contents

Throughout the book, I have personally selected oil products and supplements to support your system during this process. Do your due diligence in researching the benefits of these oils for your Keto journey.

There is a multitude of companies who make supplements and essential oils available. I have researched a myriad of companies and products before deciding which brand I will use. There is only one that I use and recommend. If you want additional training or would like to know more, reach out to me at: sharnael@swiftfire.org or DM me on social media.

Introduction

"Get off sugar!"

That is what I heard, an inner/outer voice that woke me up several nights in a row, in December 2014. I pay attention to those kinds of things, especially after the third or fourth time of hearing it within the night. Maybe you know what I am talking about spiritually. Sometimes there is this knowing, this sense that God I Am is speaking. It is something within you that you cannot get away from. I listened to the voice, but in the back of my mind I was thinking, '*I am just going to do a two or three day fast.*' I started looking around for information about fasting and eliminating sugar. I scouted Facebook for no-sugar groups and the only one I could find was a "just-say-no-to-sugar-for-a-year" type of group. I thought to myself, '*Nope, that sounds crazy... a whole year? No.*'

One night, in January 2015, I had Doug Addison[a] as a guest on my show and he was talking about setting goals and how to do it. One of the things I told him was, "Yeah, I am going to do a 3-day, get off sugar deal," and I was really excited about it. Doug, a dear friend of mine, is someone I had worked with over the years doing ministry together. We met when working with John Paul Jackson[b] years ago and have

---

a   Doug Addison is the founder and president of InLight Connection. He is a prophetic speaker, author, and coach. He is best known for his *Daily Prophetic Words* and *Spirit Connection* webcast, podcast, and blog.

b   John Paul Jackson (1950-2015) was the founder of Streams Ministries International. He was an authority on biblical dream interpretation as well as a prolific author, speaker, and teacher.

done numerous conferences together over the years. By the time I mentioned my intentions of eliminating sugar, we had already known each other and worked together over a decade. I was surprised when Doug said, "Well, you know, I have been off sugar for 10 years." His response shocked me because I did not know how anyone could be sugar-free for a year, let alone 10. Over the years I had traveled with him, so I witnessed his eating habits, but he never came out and declared that he intentionally ate a sugar-free diet. When we would go get Chinese food, he would not eat the rice, and skipped the noodles too, but again, he never announced that he was eating a carb-free diet.

It was then that I realized this person that I know and respect has been off sugar for *10 years*. I can probably handle one year.

With apprehension, I joined that Facebook group anyway. (Insert YIKES!) I committed to giving up sugar for one year. I created my own group as well, because I thought maybe some of my friends would want to do it and we could have a little bit more interaction and privacy. I lost 48 pounds in about 12 weeks, and I went on to lose a total of 103 pounds. The majority of that was due to the Ketogenic lifestyle. My friends and I were essentially practicing the Keto lifestyle; although the word 'Keto' was an unknown phenomenon at that time.

Before we begin, I just want you to know that this lifestyle is not necessarily about losing weight, but it CAN be a big part of it. You may not want to lose weight and that is fine. This is about making better choices for your body. Not only is sugar addictive, but it also causes inflammation in the body, stress on the liver, it can contribute to leptin resistance, it can increase bad cholesterol and triglycerides, and so much more.

I want to say that again simply, so you really understand: sugar is poison. There are better options for you, and I will help you work through them as you read this book. I work with all kinds of people, all at different ranges and stages of this process. You do not have to be an expert to jump in and get started.

It is important to RE-Member that Keto is a journey, not a quick-fix sprint. You will *feel* results usually in three to four days and *see* results in one to two weeks. However, just as with any other lifestyle change, it is a choice and a commitment. Sometimes it is a commitment. There is always something more to learn on this journey. Before you begin, I would like to tell you a little bit more about me.

As a Naturopathic Doctor, as well as an experienced 'Ketonian' myself, I have done a lot of research within this specific arena. Anything that I recommend is because I have personally tried it and can testify to it unless stated otherwise. Do your due diligence and research everything before you try it, to ensure it is right for you. I strongly suggest you check with your own doctor for what is best for you, personally.

How to Make Best Use of This Book

Read this book in its *entirety* first. That way, you will have all the information to see how this lifestyle works. Then when you know you are ready, get in prep-mode and start back at the beginning to begin practicing the reset now that you are equipped with the bigger picture in mind.

After you have finished your initial reading, start with one chapter a day, preferably in the morning, and use these words to RE-Mind yourself that you are choosing to balance your body by feeding it good, healthy foods and teaching it to perform better than ever.

You only get this one body on Earth, so it is important that you take care of it the best way possible. Whenever you would like some inspiration or more information about the Keto journey, just pick up the book and read a chapter to RE-Mind yourself what you need to do.

If you would like to join an online Keto community for extra support, recipes, fun, and accountability, please join mine at www.swiftfire.org/onlineclasses.

You can find more information, including how to join, in the resources section at the back of the book.

PREP-TIME SUGGESTIONS IF YOU START NOW INSTEAD OF READING THE WHOLE BOOK FIRST

1. Rid your house of sugary, 'carby' snacks.
2. Replace with meats, cheeses, and carb-free or low-carb veggies. See Day 15 for a few suggestions.
3. Your total limit per day is 10-20 carbs, so keep this in mind when looking at labels.

    Please note: carbs turn to sugar, so we are counting CARBS not sugar.
4. The day before you start, I suggest an early dinner, and then no snacks or eating **at all** until **noon** the next day, to jump-start your Ketosis process. (This is called 'intermittent fasting', or IF.)
5. If you do choose to jump in now without reading, you can join the interactive group at the discounted price. (I have videos on each of the things mentioned above, such as: snacks, shopping, reading labels and IF). This group is discounted as my gift to you. It is a great resource to compliment this book. You can find it all here: www.swiftfire.org/onlineclass. *Discount Code "KETODISCOUNT"*

Day 1:

Basics of Keto

What Is Ketosis?

I am so excited for the journey you are about to take into Ketogenics. As a Naturopathic Doctor, I know how effective and efficient the Keto lifestyle is for overall health. I did not write this book just because I know how great it is, I wrote it because my destiny is to help other people find their destinies—and your health is a big part of that.

In the past, I had some pretty serious health issues. I weighed 220 pounds and was taking 30 different medications. If that sounds familiar, then I have good news for you-a healthier life is just a few weeks away. I was able to get off all of my meds and reduce my weight drastically to 117 pounds, thanks to a lot of different reprogramming, making better choices, and doing things naturally. Keto was a major factor in that.

So, what do all these words (Ketosis, Ketogenics, Keto, etc.) really mean? Well, our bodies require fuel to do everything: to think, to eat, to pump blood through our circulatory system, even to sit and read this book. This machine we call a body requires fuel to function in any way. Most of the time, due to the modern day diet, the fuel that we use is primarily from sugar or carbohydrates (carbs).

We have an overabundant supply of sugar at our fingertips pretty much anywhere, from the grocery store, to the gas station, to the office supply store. Seriously, if you go to Office Depot right now, there will be two rows of sweets and temptation right in front of you at the checkout.

Our caveman ancestors had to gather food from the earth and kill animals to eat. There were no buffets readily available, or gas stations around the corner where you could buy sugary fuel for your body. Hunting was seasonal. Winter months were freezing cold and animals were hibernating. Luckily, our bodies were designed to store extra fat for the winter. That way, we could use fat as fuel to keep us alive and functioning. But, guess what? We do not have to hunt for our food anymore. Well, not really. Instead, we "hunt" for food at grocery or convenience stores, where we find a huge selection of food for us to purchase. Whether or not it is actual "food" that we choose is debatable. (Most are just empty and quickly digested calories that actually pull minerals from the body during digestion.) Because of this over-supply of food, we never actually tap into the fat storage in and around our bodies.

When you remove carbs/sugar as a type of fuel from your body, your body responds by looking for other ways to be fed. This is the process of going into fat adaptation. Fat adaptation is the preferred metabolic state of any human. To be in fat adaptation means your body uses its stored fat as the means for fuel and energy. Being fat-adapted is what occurred within the cavemen's bodies and there are many benefits to being in this state for us today.

At this point, the liver will respond by creating Ketones. Ketones are released into the bloodstream, looking around for stored fat to eat up and use as energy for your body. This is how you have the drive to do all the things that you are supposed to do without tiring easily.

Nutritional Ketosis is the name for this process. If you are pulling from your stored fat and breaking it down, then eventually you are going to run out of stored fat. At that point, your body will start eating into your muscles for protein. To be honest, most of us either have so much stored fat or we are eating enough good, healthy fats, that our bodies do not turn to the muscles as food. This is not something that is common, or something that should cause you any concern.

As I mentioned earlier, sugar causes inflammation. Many disease states are fed by carbs/sugar. Cancer loves sugar. Mood swings, achy joints, candida, and yeast infections—all of these things are affected by sugar. When you remove sugar, you starve those diseases and infections, so they diminish and eventually go away.

What are some of the other benefits of Ketosis?

Removing carbs/sugar helps to reset hormones. You will sleep so much better, you will think clearly, you will wake up easier, and you will find that your energy is off the charts, especially starting Day 3 or Day 4.

When I first eliminated sugar, I was cleaning my house like a crazy person because I had an incredible amount of energy. I went to bed at 9:00 p.m., got sleepy like a normal person, and woke up without an alarm clock. Ridding the body of sugar will shift your sleep patterns, it will shift your energy, and it will shift the clarity of your brain.

In the next chapter, I will discuss the effects of sugar a bit further so that you understand what a great choice you are making for your body, by eliminating it from your diet.

Day 2:

Sugar Facts

I am going to be real with you here: The American Heart Association recommends only six teaspoons a day of sugar. Unfortunately, the sugar consumption in America is incredibly high.

"In 1915, the average person consumed 15 to 20 pounds of sugar each year. Today, we consume our own bodyweight in sugar, plus 20 pounds of additional corn syrup. There is an average of $54 billion in the dental industry right now because of tooth decay from sugar consumption." Sugar is **everywhere**.

I stopped drinking soda in 2009 because soda is one of the biggest culprits of sugar intake. If the goal is between 10 and 20 carbs per day, but a 12-ounce can of soda with 39 grams of sugar is consumed daily, that is already way past the daily limit of carbs. I have had clients who were drinking a couple of *liters* of soda each day! Yikes! It is a well-known fact that soda has a ton of carbs/sugar and is terrible for us. Drink water.

What about coffee?

Coffee is great. However, one grande, white chocolate mocha from Starbucks with nonfat milk and no whip has 56 grams of sugar in it. That is five days worth of the daily carb limit if you follow the 10/20 carb rule. Wendy's green tea has 33 carbs. I am not saying this to knock restaurants, but to help you become more mindful about what you are choosing. There are some things, like green tea or a non-fat mocha, that you might think is a healthy choice, but it is really a poor choice. Look out for hidden sugars as well, because even if all those green juices in the supermarket look clean and healthy, the carb count will tell you the truth. The numbers do not lie.

Drinks are not the only things that contain hidden sugars. Take eggs. At a local diner one day, I merely ordered eggs. I thought eggs seemed "safe," but for some reason I got kicked out of Ketosis. I could not figure out why? I mean…*eggs?!* I went back to the restaurant and asked more about the menu when I discovered that the people who were cooking the food were not giving me *real eggs*; they were actually using *powdered eggs*, which is mixed with milk and who knows what else?

We have to ask if what we are getting is real food or packaged food. Also, anything white will have carbs/sugar: potatoes, pasta, cereal, pancakes, cookies, cakes, etc. All of those 'foods' contain carbs. Just be careful because there may be things that you are eating every day that you do not realize contain sugar or carbs.

When you remove sugar from the equation, you are going to feel so much better in every area of your life. Removing this one ingredient will affect everything including cholesterol, blood sugar, mood swings, emotional ups and downs, and will ease joint movement.

There is an addictive side to sugar, too. Sugar affects your brain. There is an increasing body of research that tells us sugar can be as addictive as some street drugs and have similar effects on the brain. Sugar literally alters the brain's chemistry. When we eat sugar, opioids and dopamine are released.

"Research shows that sugar can be even more addicting than cocaine," says Cassie Bjork, R.D., L.D., founder of Healthy Simple Life. "Sugar activates the opiate receptors in our brain and affects the reward center, which leads to compulsive behavior, despite the negative consequences like weight gain, headaches, hormone imbalances, and more."

As we eat sugar it activates the 'reward center' of our mind. The more we eat it, the better we feel, then we repeat. This causes a habitual and chemical "need" to get that "high."

This is why I recommend a <u>minimum</u> 21-day plan to start. It is way better to do 31 days just to reinforce things, but if we can change the program, detoxify, and do a minimum of 21 days, we can alter the pathways in the brain to create new paths, new habits, and a new chemistry.

From a neuroscience perspective, we are literally deprogramming; RE-Minding, reprogramming, and RE-Membering.

If this is different than what you are used to, I invite you to try it out, at least for your first 21 to 31 days. I will walk you through this naturally, without ANY artificial supplements.

Day 3:

Exogenous vs. Nutritional Ketosis and Ketone Supplements

It is important in the beginning to clarify that I am _not_ talking about _exogenous_ Ketosis. Exogenous by definition means: originating externally, manufactured, synthetic.

Your body will go into Ketosis on its own without synthetic help.

Exogenous Ketones are not created from the body. There are Ketone supplements out there, however I will not discuss those in any part of this book and do not recommend them at all!

The focus here, is on _nutritional_ Ketosis, meaning the Ketones your own body creates, not the kind you buy over the counter. There is not enough research to tell people all of the health risks of exogenous Ketosis, but I can tell you that I have seen several dozen bad cases already on my own.

If you use supplements to induce Ketosis, you are just drinking or eating a lot of synthetic Ketones and then eliminating them when you 'pee.' When you use the testing sticks, they show when you "have Ketones" in your urine, but _that is not your body creating them._ (More on Keto sticks in a future chapter.)

If you are taking supplements it will appear that you are in Ketosis, but you will find that the minute you stop taking the supplements, the urine test will show that is no longer the case.

When participating in *nutritional* Ketosis, meaning eliminating sugar and allowing your own body to make Ketones for you, a metabolism shift occurs. You first create the Ketones, then the Ketones go throughout your body. That is how actual nutritional Ketosis transpires.

I tried Ketone supplements for a few days as a test with some colleagues, as did some of my clientele. Big mistake. Some of the supplement brands advertise that you can eat whatever you want and still remain in Ketosis. What I discovered was that this claim was far from the truth. I ate whatever I wanted one day and took the Ketone supplements to 'stay in Ketosis.' When I tested, it showed I was in Ketosis. I thought, *"Oh, good, I stayed in Ketosis! That is great. I screwed up, but I took the supplements and they kept me going along. I will be fine tomorrow."* Well, the next day, I was not 'fine.'

Any medicine you take makes a similar claim. If you take a thyroid medication, your thyroid will say, *"I do not need to do this on my own because someone is doing it for me,"* and it will stop working on its own. I took those supplements as a test, with three other doctors experimenting with me. It took four weeks for my body to make Ketones on its own again, and I actually gained weight.

My kidneys were taxed because of it too. They were working so hard to get the synthetic Ketones out because they saw them as foreign objects.

Your body is meant to make its own Ketones, not have them added artificially. It is extremely dangerous, because your kidneys and liver are not meant to have high levels of sugar, insulin, *and* supplement-based Ketones in your body. The liver's whole process of making Ketones is what makes your body dip into its own fat stores. THIS is what changes the metabolism.

It is worth repeating again: do not take any kind of Ketone supplements.

Encouraging the body to produce energy, balance, and transmute weight on its own—gradually and without unnecessary supplementation—is best. Taking short cuts usually does not pay off in the long run and could be more harmful to you.

If you are interested in getting your body into a state of Ketosis, I encourage you to do it through your diet and lifestyle change.

Want the best tricks for getting into (and staying in) full Ketosis? Keep reading.

Day 4:

Keto and Reading Labels

What I will not tell you, is what you can and cannot eat, because I am not your mama. I want this to be your choice. I do not want to take anything away from you, because when you are denied something, there is sometimes a ripple effect of needing it more, or feeling further tempted to get it. I *am* asking you, however, to stick with a maximum of 10 to 20 carbs a day.

Personally, since 2014, I have stayed between 10 and 15 carbs daily. Yes, there have been times when I was not in Ketosis, either on purpose or accidentally, which resulted in me getting kicked out of Ketosis. I know that it is doable, and that it is not harmful. I am asking you to start out with 10 to 20 carbs a day ideally, for the next 21 to 31 days.

This really helps your body and brain to detoxify and reprogram.

Reading labels is a skill that is really necessary for Keto, because the key to Keto is eating very low carbs. You cannot do that if you do not know how many carbs are hiding in a food or product.

The first thing you are going to look for is the carb count. We need to count carbs. Once you see the total number of carbs on the label, you can subtract any *fiber* or *sugar alcohols*. (You can subtract sugar alcohols because they will not induce insulin or cause you to stop releasing Ketones.) Ramen packets, for example, contain about 26 grams of carbohydrates; they only have one gram of fiber, so that would be 25 total carbs! That is more than the suggested daily carb count.

The other thing you need to be careful about is the *serving size*. Items like pre-bottled smoothies that appear to be single-servings can actually contain more than one serving. What you are looking at on the label is what one serving contains, when the entire bottle may contain multiple servings. Most foods have way more carbs than you might think. Macaroni and cheese is one example. I did some research and found that a box of macaroni and cheese has 47 grams of carbs and 2 grams of fiber, giving us a total count of 45 carbohydrates. WOW! And... often people ask me if gluten-free carbohydrates are better, so I looked at a box of gluten-free macaroni and cheese and, guess what? There were 48 total grams of carbohydrates in one serving. MORE?!

Once, I was staying at a hotel and I ordered an omelet at their restaurant. I saw the cook in the back literally pull a frozen omelet out of the freezer and pop it in the microwave, already folded and everything. *(Side note: Get rid of your microwave; radiation is harmful and no one needs it in their home[c].)* The other eggs that they were making were not 'real' eggs either; they were out of a carton. I asked, "Can you tell me if these are real eggs?" and she told me she would "check the box."

Gasp. Check the box?!

She came out a moment later with her carton and, sure enough, there were carbs in the 'box.'

They put sugar on french fries, and even in bread. Two pieces of bread is equivalent to one Snickers bar, so you might as well eat a Snickers bar if you want some bread.

---

c   Subscribe to my YouTube channel *Dr. Sharnael Wolverton Sehon* and watch my video titled *The Science of Microwaves w Dr Sharnael.*

Again, I am not telling you what to eat, but if you choose to eat all of your daily carbs in the form of Doritos, cookies or whatever and just not eat for the rest of the day, that is your choice. It is not going to be very nutritious for you and you will probably be pretty hungry. A lot of times when we feel hungry, it is really our brain saying that it requires nutrients. If you eat a bunch of food that has no nutrients in it, then guess what? You will still be hungry! There are a lot of things that have few or no carbs such as meat, chicken, or fish. Those will fill you up and make you feel much better than Doritos, *and* you can pretty much eat all you need to feel full.

I encourage you to eat real food—nothing processed, nothing boxed, and no fast food—as much as possible at least for these 31 days. Ideally, that is what we would all be doing all the time, but even I am partial to chocolate and snacks every once in a while. I want you to choose whole, raw foods and prepare them so that you can see how much better you feel when you put good fuel in your body.

I also recommend a glass of warm water in the morning before you have anything else. Add some fresh lemon or Vitality™ essential oils, and drink this first thing upon waking. You may also want to get a water bottle of some kind to keep next to your bed.

Finally, I recommend fasting for the first day. I am an all-or-nothing person, so I like to only eat between the hours of noon through dinner time, which is called intermittent fasting. That has been a very quick way for me to get into good eating habits. Intermittent fasting, or IF, really speeds up the metabolism and helps because the longer you are not eating, the more the Ketones are using that fuel it has stored to run your body. We will get more into the benefits of intermittent fasting, whole foods, and lemon water as you work through the book, but try some of these ideas out in the meantime.

Reading labels is the best way for you to know exactly how many carbs you are putting into your body, so that you can monitor them and have the divine success and health of your choosing. To keep your carb count down and be able to actually measure it, RE-Member this formula: **Carbs – fiber – sugar alcohols = your net carbs per serving**. Try to stick with the 10-20 carb daily limit, especially for this short time.

Get a food diary or journal and write down what you are eating each day, so you can really keep track of your success. Once you start reading labels, you may be surprised at the number of items that contain hidden sugar. I provide a list in the next chapter.

Day 5:

120 Names for Sugar

Time to talk about sugars and sweeteners. By now, you should instinctively be turning over labels to read the ingredients. Sugar can hide in foods and you may not even know it. The list below contains 120 different names that manufacturers use to conceal sugar. Definitely stay away from these!

Be wary of "sugar-free" or "no sugar added" claims on products, as well. There are many sugar substitutes that can still cause a spike in insulin response and kick you out of Ketosis. Some of these are: aspartame (Nutrisweet, Equal), sucralose (Splenda), maltodextrin, maltitol, dextrose, acesulfame potassium (Ace-k). These can also cause stomach and digestive track irritation, diarrhea, and bloating for some people.

Agave Nectar
Amazake
Anhydrous
   Dextrose
Barbados Sugar
Bark Sugar
Barley Malt
Barley Malt Syrup
Beet Sugar
Blackstrap Molasses

Brown Rice Syrup
Brown Sugar
Buttered Syrup
Cane Juice
Cane Juice Crystals
Cane Sugar
Caramel
Carbitol
Carob Syrup
Castor Sugar

Coconut Palm
   Sugar
Coconut Sugar
Confectioner's
   Sugar
Corn Sweetener
Corn Syrup
Corn Syrup Solids
Crystal Dextrose
Crystalline Fructose

D-tagatose
Date Sugar
Dehydrated Cane Juice
Demerara Sugar
Dextran
Dextrin
Dextrose
Diastatic Malt
Diatase
Diglycerides
Disaccharides
Ethyl Maltol
Florida Crystals
FOS (fructo-oligosaccharides)
Fructose
Fructose Sweetener
Fruit Juice
Fruit Juice Concentrate
Galactose
Glucitol
Glucosamine
Gluconolactone
Glucose
Glucose Solids
Glycerides
Glycerine
Glycerol
Glycol
Golden Sugar
Golden Syrup
Grape Sugar
HFCS (high-fructose corn syrup)
Hexitol
Honey
Icing Sugar
Inversol
Isomalt
Invert Sugar
Jaggery
Karo Syrup
Lactose
Levulose
Liquid Fructose
Malitol
Malt Syrup
Malted Barley
Malts
Maltodextrin
Maltose
Mannitol
Mannose
Maple Syrup
Microcrystalline Cellulose
Molasses
Monoglycerides
Monosaccharides
Muscovado
Nectars
Organic Raw Sugar
Palm Sugar
Pancake Syrup
Panocha
Pentose
Polydextrose
Polyglycerides
Powdered Sugar
Raisin Juice
Raisin Syrup
Raw Sugar
Refiner's Syrup
Ribose Rice Syrup
Rice Malt
Rice Sugar
Rice Syrup
Rice Syrup Solids
Rice Sweeteners
Saccharides
Sorbitol
Sorghum
Sorghum Syrup
Sucanat
Sucrose
Sweet Sorghum
Syrup
Treacle
Trisaccharides
Turbinado Sugar
Unrefined Sugar
White Sugar
Yellow Sugar
Zylose

So what can you have? Look for products with the following Keto-approved sweeteners. These typically do not cause an insulin response or have adverse effects. As always, only use them in moderation!

STEVIA (all natural, plant-based)

MONK FRUIT (all natural, plant-based)

ERYTHRITOL (all natural, fermented from corn sources, the easiest of the sugar alcohols to digest)

XYLITOL (can be used to prevent tooth decay, natural, usually derived from birch wood; NOTE: toxic to dogs!)

Staying away from sugars, carbs, and processed foods will help your body stay in Ketosis. The best way to know if your body is functioning in Ketosis properly is to test your urine or your blood. In the next chapter, I will teach you about the best testing method and what it means.

Day 6:

The Keto Sticks

Keto sticks are a great tool to measure how many Ketones are in your body. They are a fast, accurate, and reliable way to determine whether you are actually in Ketosis.

When Ketones are released into the body through the bloodstream, those Ketones eventually exit the body through urination. That is how you will know for sure that you are truly in Ketosis. There are sticks that you can urinate on to measure your Ketones; brand names such as ReliOn and Ketostix which are available at any pharmacy like Rite Aid, Walgreens, or CVS, just to name a few. These sticks are either behind the counter, or they may be in the diabetic health section as a lot of people use them to check for diabetes or hypoglycemia.

You can also order them online, just be aware of the expiration date written on the box. I have accidentally purchased expired batches, and have tested several times with an expired batch, because I was not aware of the expiration. Once the package is open, that is when the first day starts. I like to write the date that I opened them on the top of the container with a sharpie. Try it! That way you know you have a certain amount of time to use them.

To save money, you can cut the sticks lengthwise down the middle with scissors to make twice the amount. Refill the empty bottles to keep one in your bag, one in the bathroom, and one at work. That way, you always have them on hand. I like to test two or three times a day, so I even keep one in my car!

Now that you have an idea about what type of sticks you need, I will discuss how to use them. First, you know that it is the liver that releases Ketones into your bloodstream. Keto sticks were developed to measure the number of Ketones that pass into your urine. Go to the bathroom and urinate on one of the sticks. It will indicate the degree to which you are releasing Ketones. In the beginning, you will only release a small amount of Ketones, but it will get higher over time. When you get into the second and third day of full Ketogenesis, you will release some of the Ketones into your urine.

My recommendation is that you begin testing as soon as possible, so that you can not only practice with the sticks, but also so you can see what it looks like when you are in the low to negative zone for Ketone release. That way, as your body continues to let go of more and more, you will be able to really see the progress and know that cutting out the carbs and the sugar has actually created a response. I do not know about you, but I like reinforcement and rewards. It encourages me to know I have accomplished my goals; knowing and feeling the instant gratification that I have actually done something. The sticks give you immediate results. Having something measurable that I can actually see keeps me motivated to continue working on creating better habits.

It is not until the first 48 to 72 hours have passed that you really start seeing the Ketones. Why is that? Well, your body is working through a process. If you suddenly have an influx of Ketones in your body, your kidneys are not going to be happy about that. Your body goes into Ketosis slowly because the kidneys have to get used to RE-Membering how to flush them out, and how to keep up with the additional work.

Similar to the exogenous Ketone supplements that we talked about, taking them will cause your kidneys to become overwhelmed quickly, which they are not prepared to handle because they did not get that adjustment period to regulate. Artificial supplements could even cause some damage in your kidneys and liver because those organs are not used to that level of Ketone release. The supplemental Ketones are foreign to the body; they are not real so the body does not know what to do with them. Exogenous means they are made outside of the body. Endogenous means they are made naturally inside your body.

By the third or fourth day, you should be in full Ketosis. I like to use these sticks to make sure I am staying in the right zone. I prefer to be in the upper-middle level because, if I accidentally ingest sugar, it is not going to immediately kick me out of Ketosis.

It is also important to drink a lot of water so you are flushing them out. Every time you cheat, or every time you have an issue where sugar or carbs sneak into something that you ate, you have to start completely over with the three to four day process. I hope you choose to use them as well, for motivation and gratification on your Keto adventure.

This journey will change your life, but only if you allow it. If you fully buy into the Keto lifestyle and move past any potential discomfort, you will acquire the results you sought out from the beginning.

Day 7:

Keto Flu

Every now and again I have had someone ask me about a phenomenon called the *'Keto flu.'* It is not something the average person knows about, but anyone who has done some research has probably come across the phrase. While it sounds scary, it is just a natural process of beginning Ketosis. <u>Sometimes</u> people (not everyone) experience it in the first two to five days that they are eliminating sugar.

As we discussed earlier, a big reason for this is because sugar is *incredibly* addictive. Medical professionals have done brain scans and they have found that sugar is so addictive that it is similar to a cocaine addiction. If you are not willing to ingest cocaine every day, you should be equally wary of sugar, because it has the same effect on your brain that drugs do to make you crave them.

When you eliminate the sugar, the body and the brain start to go into withdrawal which can trigger flu-like symptoms: headaches, achy joints, low-grade temperature, even mood swings. The candida and yeast that are present in the body can make you crave sugar even more as you begin to eliminate it from your diet, because sugar is what feeds those things. Eliminating sugar starves them. Also, sugar gives the brain a shot of dopamine and the brain is used to getting that, so it starts looking for new ways to make dopamine.

Your body may also experience some issues with Keto flu because it has been using sugar for fuel. Now, without that fuel, you require more enzymes to break down fat and convert it with the Ketones. Ketones are now converting your own fat into the fuel the body needs to function. With that need for more enzymes, it is really helpful to eat a more plant-based diet, because plants are loaded with great enzymes.

In the past, our food was grown differently and had a lot more natural enzymes than it does today. I encourage you to take enzymes to help your body become more efficient. My favorite one is Essentialzymes™. I take it with meals and in between meals, and I recommend that you find some enzymes you can take to aid your healthy body in this process as well.

Another reason why your body may experience the Keto flu is because it is detoxing. Fat actually holds onto chemicals and toxins. When you are using any kind of chemicals—bleaches and shampoos, room sprays, insect sprays, perfumes etc.—your body absorbs any chemicals you ingest or that come in contact with your skin. Your body then stores them in your fat to prevent those chemicals from entering your bloodstream. When you start melting your fat with the Ketones, these toxins are being released into your bloodstream and they are looking to get out.

In order to help any of these symptoms that your body might be experiencing, I highly recommend WATER! I also recommend exercise, which creates endorphins and dopamine that can be really helpful to support the transition. Stretching is very good for the body too. There are some great stretches that are helpful for resetting the brain and the body's electrical system. A chemical called Christos is released from the pituitary and the pineal gland. Christos goes into your body's electrical system, down the spine of your back, and fires off, hitting all the electrical parts of your body. Then, when it comes back up, it actually looks for dormant brain cells to ignite.

In addition to water, I would also like to suggest using a few different essential oils and vitamins to support your healthy body. You may consider bumping up your potassium, magnesium, and B vitamins. My personal favorite is Super B™.

There are some foods that can help fight these symptoms as well, specifically kale, avocado, and healthy greens. If you do not like these foods, you can juice them, which is my favorite way to take them in. Massages help support a healthy body as well as Raindrop Technique® and infrared sauna.

If you are feeling any of these symptoms, hang in there. I promise that you will feel so much better in just a couple days. Two days from now you will be saying how great you are feeling, how clear your brain is, and how improved your sleep has been.

Studies show that when you get into Ketosis, you actually create and sprout new brain cells! Your energy is going to be high, your brain will sharpen, and you will have a much easier time saying 'no' to all the carbs.

Day 8:

What Is Candida and
What's It Got to Do with Keto?

In the previous chapter, I listed candida as one of the reasons why someone might experience the Keto flu. Did you know that 85% of Americans have a substance called candida in their body? Candida is a yeast-like fungus that lives in and off of our bodies. Candida can be good as far as helping to aid in the absorption of nutrients and with digestion, but an overgrowth of candida is a bad thing. We need to identify whether or not we are dealing with a candida overgrowth in our bodies, and learn how to support a healthy gut and a healthy body.

Allow me to identify some of the ways to know if we are dealing with candida:

1. Whether a child or adult, if you have a thrush-like white tongue or sores in your mouth, that is candida.

2. If you are dealing with a "muffin-top" around your mid-section that you cannot seem to get rid of or release, it could be a telltale sign that you may be dealing with candida.

3. Skin issues such as rashes and itchiness, a yeast infection, and/or yellowing fingernails or toenails are also good indicators that candida may be present.

4. Children can pick up candida from the birth canal or through breast milk. Scientists have studied the umbilical cord of a child at birth and found over 200 chemicals present!

5. Brain fog, joint pain, an overall feeling of being unwell, or inflamed, chronic allergies, sinus infections, digestion problems, mood swings, UTIs, and bad immunity overall are good indicators of candida.

6. Even bad breath is another indication that you may have a candida overgrowth.

Candida is at the root of a lot of your sugar cravings as well, because sugar is what feeds it. When you start eating Keto and start eliminating carbohydrates and sugar from your diet, candida gets pretty ticked off. It starts yelling at you, "Give me that sugar! Give me those carbs!" because it is trying to survive. If you have candida, it goes into the intestine and lives there.

If you are on antibiotics or prescriptions, the candida can start breaking through the walls of your intestines and leak out into your body; a condition called "leaky gut." Then, the yeast can get into the bloodstream and cause infections, which can be dangerous.

What causes candida overgrowth? Things like birth control pills, sugar, and high-carb diets are all contributors. Alcohol is another big contributor to an overgrowth of candida. Think about the average American diet: highly processed food, high sugar food, and a lot of carbohydrates. When you see anything on a label that says low fat, you can guarantee that means they have increased the carbohydrates and upped the sugar to keep some kind of taste. Watch out for low fat anything! There as nothing wrong with fat. There are good fats that are important for your body, but those high sugar, high carb diets can speed up candida growth.

It is important to know how to support a healthy gut, because there are a lot of ways to take control of your body and create your own personal, divine health. Your health is your responsibility, and you can change your environment and your choices to treat your body the way that it deserves to be treated. Probiotics are one way to support a healthy gut. My favorite is Life 9™. Probiotics are particularly helpful for anyone who has taken antibiotics, because antibiotics kill everything—even the good stuff! There are good, important flora in your gut and antibiotics can wipe all of those out. Replacing those flora is important.

You can drink kefir, kombucha, or any other probiotic drink. My favorite is Kevita, but when you can drink anything like Kevita—especially the lower carb Kevita flavors such as lemon, tangerine lemon, lemon cayenne, and even hibiscus—they only have one or two carbs, and they are delicious and packed with probiotics. RE-Member to look at the carbs and the sugar, because you do not want to get probiotics at the expense of adding a lot of sugar to your diet.

Bentonite clay is another thing you can try. I have not used that personally, but I have heard a lot of different people who have experienced really good results.

Slique® tea is great support for a healthy gut. It is low-carb, good for you, and tasty.

Coconut oil is another awesome choice. You can have a spoonful of this every day or more, if you choose, or put it in your coffee. Coconut kills candida and it tastes pretty good.

You should also consider adding vitamin C to your diet. Super C™ is my favorite because it is a chewable tablet and my body does not have to digest it as much. It is packed with good-for-you stuff, including rosehip, citrus, and cherry. It tastes really good, is high in vitamin C, and the kids love it too.

Another great support product for your healthy body system is ParaFree™. Do your due diligence on this. I love this product.

I love balance, so I hope this has been helpful for you. Again, 85% of Americans are on a high-level sugar diet. You make choices every day about what you put in your mouth. That alone is going to do some great things for you, so consider joining a Keto group or connecting with people who are using Keto, because that is a great way to completely change a lot of different things in your body for the better. Finally, a Keto way of life is going to be helpful for a lot of reasons besides the increased energy, fat burning, mental clarity, and better sleep, because it will starve out the overabundance of candida in your body.

The fact that you have this book and have made the choice to follow the Keto lifestyle means that you have already taken the first steps toward embracing and supporting your own divine health. God has given us some great tools, such as plants, that He has provided for our benefit.

I have mentioned intermittent fasting a few times in this book already, and the next chapter is devoted to how much it can help your body. It is a simple change that will take your results to the next level when living Keto.

If you choose to do so, flip to the end of this book and check out my resources. I have listed some groups and resources that can be supportive and helpful for you as you begin this new lifestyle change.

Day 9:

Candida Spit Test

Here is a little more candida information for you: the spit test. This is an easy test that will help you determine if candida is an issue for you.

Candida lives in your intestinal tract and affects the digestive system, but it can come up your esophagus and into your mouth. That is how we can test the spit to determine if you have a candida overgrowth.

How does the test work? Get a glass of water and put it next to your bed. When you first wake up in the morning, immediately spit into the glass. Wait three minutes and then look at your spit. If it gets stringy and starts falling, sinks like an anchor, or gets really cloudy, then you are probably dealing with some candida overgrowth in your body.

If your test comes out positive, please do not worry! Flip back to the candida chapter to see what you can do to limit and eradicate some of the candida overgrowth in your body. Again, 85% of Americans deal with candida, so, more likely than not, it is something you will have to correct in your own body.

Many people try to tell themselves that the reason they do not practice Keto is because it is too restrictive. That is really not true. The next few chapters will show you that there are *a lot* of delicious treats that you can enjoy.

Day 10:

Intermittent Fasting

I am providing this advice with years of experience, knowledge, and education under my belt. Intermittent fasting (IF) is **so** good for the body. I have been fasting off and on for years as both a spiritual practice as well as for the health benefits. We did not call it intermittent fasting back then, we just called it fasting.

Did you know that IF can slow the aging process? It detoxifies your body by getting rid of all the chemicals, pharmaceuticals, and foreign substances in your system; things like food coloring, MSG, and all that other stuff that we do not want hanging around. IF also ramps up your energy! Who does not need energy in this day and age? Everyone I know could use a little boost. Intermittent fasting taps into the fat storage of your body and converts the fat into Ketones, which helps to burn more fat, and that is exactly what we are choosing to do with eating Keto!

Fasting also increases the levels of human growth hormone (HGH) in your body, which means it lowers cholesterol, and repairs damaged DNA, skin, and the lining of your stomach. When we go to sleep, our body produces HGH, releasing it into our body to help the healing and restoration process. Dr. Gary Young always told us, 'The highest levels of HGH are released between 10:00 p.m. to midnight." This is why I recommend that people sleep more than they probably are. Sleeping is beneficial, especially in that 10 p.m. to midnight period. If you can sleep during those two hours, it is like you are getting four hours of sleep instead of just two.

Human growth hormone is critical for repairing our DNA and cells, so when you combine it with fasting, the window for the time that you are releasing HGH is extended. When that time is extended, guess what? More time for healing! So whether or not you are sleeping, that process keeps going, and HGH is released because there is no food to digest. If you are the type to go to bed right after eating, then your body will actually be forced to choose between restoring your body or digesting the food in your stomach. If you have eaten and gone to bed on a full stomach, then your body will always pick digestion, which means you do not release HGH and you are not truly resting, so what is the point? If you choose to go to sleep on an empty stomach, however, your body will release the HGH and when you wake up while fasting, your body continues releasing HGH.

A lot of us grew up with the myth that skipping breakfast slows down our metabolism, but that is simply not true. Your metabolism does not slow down unless you have done a fast with no food at all for over 72 hours. That is a bigger difference than just missing breakfast, right? If you simply skip breakfast in the morning, studies have proven that you actually increase your metabolism up to 10 percent more. Not only do you increase your metabolism to burn more fat, but you are also keeping that extension of HGH, so you stay in repair mode even when you are awake and walking around. I think that is pretty awesome!

At this point you may be wondering what *intermittent* fasting is and what it is all about, especially because there are already so many types of fasts out there: 40-day fasts, three-day fasts, liquid fasts, juice cleanses, or the Daniel Fast, which is just vegetables. There are a lot of different types, and I am encouraging you to look into them so you can actually customize whatever kind of fast that you prefer. The point of intermittent fasting is that you take blocks of time where you are not eating as opposed to fasting all day. I encourage fasting period. You choose what's best for you.

I am going to talk about three types of fasts. One is called the Monday-Wednesday-Friday intermittent fast, which means you do not eat on Monday, Wednesday, or Friday. You do eat on the opposite days and, as long as you are eating healthy, you will see results.

There is also a 12-to-12 variation that works like this: You quit eating every night at 8 p.m., and then start back up 12 hours later at 8 a.m. Most people are probably doing that anyway, so I do not think it is difficult or asking too much in this case.

Personally, I do a 16–8 fast. That means I fast for 16 hours and have an 8-hour eating window. Here is what that looks like: if you stop eating at 8:00 p.m., then you will not eat again until noon the following day. I prefer that method because it extends my HGH production for several more hours, and it is not a difficult change to make. It is really just skipping breakfast!

If you follow an exercise regimen, there are two ways to make it work with IF. You can work out right before you start the fast in order to extend it, so you are burning through the night. For example, if you are doing the 16-8 fast and you start your fast at 8 p.m., you could work out from 7 to 8, so you are burning through the night. That does not work for everyone, because some people get so hyped up when they work out that they do not sleep well.

That leaves you with the other option - fasting until noon, but working out at 11 a.m. Many people cannot do that because they work 9-5 jobs, but in a perfect world, that would be the ideal workout situation. If you get up at 6 a.m. to work out and you still do not eat until noon, that is still going to be better for you than not working out or not fasting, because you will still have increased metabolism. The best option is to put your workout at the beginning or end of your fast, but as long as you are getting a workout in, that is what matters.

As a review, IF is not a requirement of the Keto lifestyle. If you are choosing to lose weight or to participate in a program to increase the benefits of Ketosis, however, then intermittent fasting is a beneficial practice that is good for the body. In the next chapter, I will describe another daily practice that will help you see greater results during your Keto experience.

Day 11:

Benefits of Drinking Lemon Water Daily

Since I just told you about the benefits of intermittent fasting, I would like to follow that up with a similar train of thought regarding the benefits of drinking lemon water first thing in the morning. If you choose to follow the intermittent fasting plan along with eating Keto, then I highly recommend that you begin your day with a glass of warm lemon water.

There are several health benefits and a lot of science behind this. Before I dive into those I would like to specify that, if you are using Lemon Vitality™ essential oil instead of a real lemon, then you should be drinking this out of a glass or ceramic mug, because hot water can break down any plastics and we do not want to add more chemicals to our bodies when we are working so hard to detox and eliminate them through our diet and fasting plans.

So, why do I think lemon oil or lemon water in the morning is so important?

1. Lemon water has a ton of health benefits, primarily with digestion. Your digestive process is tied in with the metabolism of the liver, so if you can detox the liver it will help jumpstart that process. The

liver will function more effectively when it is cleaned out, which is incredibly helpful while maintaining a Keto diet.

2. Lemon water can help flush those chemicals out of your fat stores, which keeps them out of your blood and keeps you feeling healthy.

3. Lemon water helps with your pH balance support—that is a pretty simple explanation, but healthy pH levels are extremely important, especially for women.

4. Lemon water balances sodium levels, which is really helpful for those of us who are not careful with our sodium intake.

5. Lemon water lowers uric acid levels.

6. Lemon water is a great source of vitamin C, which we all need, especially in the winter. Guinea pigs and humans do not create their own vitamin C, so we have to get it from outside sources, and lemon water is an excellent source.

7. Lemon water is a great source of collagen, which is good for the skin, bones, ligaments, muscles, blood vessels, and heart.

8. Lemons are high in antioxidants, which are really important in the body, especially when we are dealing with free radicals. Free radicals are **not** good for the body. They damage the cellular DNA, and can be a major cause of disease. Lemon water helps fight them.

9. Lemon water helps block cortisol levels. Cortisol is a stress chemical; it kicks in during the fight-or-flight response. A constant, high-level of stress can wreak havoc on your body, but flavonoids, which are present in lemon water, can combat the cortisol.

Just a mug of warm lemon water in the morning has all of these incredible benefits!

WHY LEMON ESSENTIAL OILS OVER LEMONS?

While many may think they are the same thing, they are not. They may taste similar, but lemon oils are cold-pressed from the rind, whereas lemon juice comes from the pulp. Essential oils are extremely concentrated and a couple of drops go a LONG way. One lemon tree can produce between 500 to 600 pounds of lemons a year, and it takes 45 lemons to fill a 15ml bottle of essential oils. Another important distinction is that essential oil may be easier to ingest for people with sensitive stomachs, because it does not contain citric acid.

Scientifically, lemon oil is higher in limonene than juice. Limonene is not only a powerful antioxidant, but also a powerful cleansing agent. It also supports a healthy respiratory function and provides immune system support, especially during seasonal changes.

I caution you to be careful. Back when I worked in restaurants, I have seen what happens when customers ask for a lemon. People think they are doing so well by putting lemon in their water, but restaurants are not always super careful with cleaning and cutting their lemons. They might let them sit out all night, or not be cleaned properly. When you order lemon water, they might just dump some of those old, unclean lemons in there, and you could be drinking everything that is on the outside of the lemon and on the rind: chemicals, mold, cleaning solution, etc. I prefer to bring my own lemons or use some sort of lemon oil.

Besides that, if you use lemon essential oils, you will get a lot more for your money, it is easier to travel with, and lemon oil is concentrated so you do not have to carry around and cut up a bunch of lemons just to get one drop. I do not personally ask for lemons when I go to restaurants, I just use my own.

That is all you need to do. Buy fresh, organic lemons or lemon essential oil, and steep them in a glass or ceramic mug full of steaming hot water. Drink up and feel amazing!

In the next chapter, I will discuss another crucial practice that you should consider including in your Keto journey: exercise. The *best* thing about all these tips I am sharing is that they work together to improve your overall health.

Day 12:

Keto and Exercise

I know not everyone is excited about exercise, particularly if you do not currently have an exercise plan, but there are just too many benefits to not mention it in relation to Ketosis.

Exercise is so important for your body, and not just in terms of maintaining a healthy weight. Exercise improves brain and memory function as well. Studies have shown with just a 20-minute walk, you can improve your brain and memory function. Just like with intermittent fasting, you can actually create and sprout new brain cells. Exercise also helps with memory, because it actually works out parts of your brain, such as the cells responsible for learning and memory.

Exercise improves your sleep patterns, allowing you to fall asleep faster and wake up easier. As you exercise and increase your circulation, you are also helping to move out some of the toxins that are being broken down by the Ketosis process happening inside your body.

Our bodies are extremely addicted to sugar, and one of the most effective ways to treat addiction is to replace an unhealthy choice with a healthy choice. If you choose to eliminate sugar, you can replace the addiction you had to the sugar-induced dopamine rush with the endorphins you get from exercise.

Of course, exercise burns calories and helps to burn fat, but the best news is, that combined with Ketosis, your body burns fat longer because your metabolism is increased so even when your body is at rest, you are still burning fat. If you want to lose weight, this is an excellent way to do just that.

Even if you do not like to exercise, there are some fun, easy ways to get those health benefits. You can take a 20-minute walk to release endorphins and dopamine throughout the day. I suggest that you work out three or four days a week, whether you take an exercise class, ride your bike, roller skate, swim, or run on a treadmill. If at all possible, I recommend getting outside as much as you can. I know that is not always possible for those of you who live in a place where it gets to -30° F outside, but that vitamin D is so good for you when you can get it. Again, exercise is not just about weight loss. It is a crucial activity that helps the body in so many areas. I ask that you choose to reach your best, most Divine Self by engaging in some form of exercise every week.

In the next few chapters I am going to give you some tips that will make your Keto process a little easier.

Day 13:

Keto Grocery Tips

Another topic I'd like to help you with in beginning the Keto lifestyle is the grocery list. In particular, it can be overwhelming figuring out what to buy or how much it will cost. I want to alleviate your concerns by giving you a few items that you can rely on as staples in your diet. The simplest change you can make is to shop <u>around the edges</u> of the grocery store, because most of what is in the middle is pre-packaged and full of preservatives and carbs! Those boxes might say things like "protein" and "fiber," but they are not the whole, real foods that are going to support your divine health. I Invite you to overcome convenience foods and make some good, healthy choices.

You know what is easy? EATING. REAL. FOOD.

Start with green vegetables, which should always be on your list. We do not have a lot of picky eaters in my family, so my typical list includes asparagus, brussel sprouts, leafy greens, cabbage, and zucchini. We make a lot of salads, lettuce wraps, and zucchini noodles with those ingredients. I also buy a lot of cauliflower, because I like to rice it or roast it. Radishes are a great alternative to potatoes; sometimes we roast or fry them.

Moving on to meats, I like to keep a lot of uncured bacon around because I fry it up and add it to my meals and then I use the bacon grease for cooking. I also prefer to buy uncured lunch meats for my family (we tend to purchase the Applegate brand). I also buy whatever meat is on sale for the week. That might be chicken, hamburger, or pork chops. I like to stock up on meat and put it in my freezer to make it last longer. Whole chickens, in particular, are something I stock up on because I like to make my own bone broth in the Instant Pot.

When you move on to the dairy section, your staples should be heavy cream, cream cheese, grass-fed butter (Kerrygold is a great brand), and sour cream. An important thing to note: buy your cheese in blocks and not pre-shredded. Most packaged shredded cheese has potato starch in it, to keep the cheese from sticking together. That potato starch adds carbs to your diet, which we do not really want when we are doing Keto, so it is easier to buy blocks of cheese and grate them yourself. I always have parmesan cheese or parmesan shavings on hand. I often make a quick sauce out of heavy cream, garlic, and parmesan to serve over zucchini noodles, chicken, or even fish. Eggs are also a major staple for my family because they are a great source of healthy fats and proteins. I usually boil eggs at the beginning of the week to use for my lunches each day.

I typically stay away from the frozen section, but there are a few healthy options you can get. I buy 100% Angus beef hamburger patties to keep in the freezer for a quick weeknight meal. I also stock up on frozen vegetables, but only those that are out of season. It is really important to eat fresh, local vegetables and meat as often as possible because those are much better for you. Stock up when your grocery staples go on sale, and avoid packaged foods.

If you are someone who enjoys alcohol occasionally, make sure you read the next chapter. I talk about how alcohol impacts the body and how it specifically relates to your Keto lifestyle.

Day 14:

Keto and Alcohol

I want to preface this section with a confession: I do not drink that much. Especially now that I have started wearing Hematite (More on this in the Crystal chapter. I also invite you to join my *Crystals, Oils, and Energy Group*[d] for more info on the science of all that.) Using this particular crystal shifted my energy, my taste buds changed completely and I just cannot tolerate the taste anymore. So many people have asked me about Keto and alcohol, however, so I included it in the book to share some information with you. I have experience with how alcohol affects the body, so I will be honest with you about a few things.

First, if your intention on this Keto journey is to eat around 10 to 20 carbs a day, know that some people do save up those carbs so they can have a glass of wine in the evening. However, there is a difference in the way carbs work in your body versus actual fuel for alcohol. The alcohol will be processed first. There is no storage unit for alcohol in the body AND your body sees alcohol as toxic poison, so it rushes to clear this out first. You may be limiting carbs, but alcohol *competes with Ketone creation and fat burning*. If you are doing 10 to 20 carbs per day and you use six of it for alcohol, those six carbs will not be counted exactly the same.

---

d   Class information can be found at www.swiftfire.org/onlineclasses

The liver produces Ketones, so if you are taking in alcohol, your liver sees it as a toxin. Your liver will prioritize getting toxicity out of the body, so it spends a lot of energy toward cleansing and detoxing itself instead of creating more Ketones and/or burning fat, which is what some people would rather be doing.

The whole thing about Ketosis is that, instead of eating or using fuel from sugar and carbs to get your body going, it will use your own fat. If you are drinking alcohol, however, it is going to burn the alcohol first, so the Ketosis may stall for a bit. Is that worth it to you? You may not be trying to lose weight, so a stall and a quick turn to burn alcohol instead of fat may not be a bad trade-off for you. It just depends on who you are and what goals you have chosen.

If you are choosing to participate in a Keto lifestyle to actually burn your own fat right now, then this may not be the choice for you.

You do not have to be on this Keto journey to lose weight. It is a great lifestyle for just the health and energy benefits alone. The good news is that once the alcohol is burned, you go straight back into creating Ketones and burning fat. You will probably never actually leave Ketosis, you are just going to switch from burning alcohol back into Ketosis. It is not like you have to start over. I have seen some people who drink and they are just fine.

Take a look at the different kinds of drinking, because if you are drinking fancy cocktails that include carbs and sugar, those will knock you out of Ketosis. On a chemistry level, your brain will have some problems because your body is going to latch onto that sugar. There are zero-carb alcoholic drinks out there which include whiskey, vodka, gin, rum, brandy, scotch, and tequila—as long as they are <u>not flavored</u>.

With beer, you are going to be imbibing at least 5 to 10 carbs for even some of the best low-carb beers out there. Rolling Rock and Michelob Ultra are the best choices for low-carb beers.

White wine ranges anywhere from 10 to 12 carbs, depending on the sugar content. Obviously a sweeter wine is going to have more sugar. Red wines sit at around 3.7 carbs. There are low-carb drinking options, you just have to be careful about what you are mixing in with them.

In all honesty, drinking alcohol shuts down the part of your brain responsible for making good decisions, and it can cause you to make some bad choices. I know people in our Keto Group who have testified some of their own mistakes. For example, they have been drinking and decided, "Hey, I will go out and have a beer with some Keto pizza." Because that part of the brain got shut down, they ended up **not** having Keto pizza. They end up getting **real** pizza and thinking it will just happen that *one time*, but just one time *will* kick you out of Ketosis. Doing this starts you over needing 72 hours to get back into Ketosis.

Another thing to think about is that, because you have not been eating high carb foods, the alcohol will affect you more than it normally would. It will go straight into your bloodstream and, since you have not been eating so many carbs, there is nothing to slow the absorption rate.

There is no reason why you have to change *everything* about your life to stay in Ketosis. The key here, as is always the case with alcohol, is to *indulge in moderation.*

You are getting so close to the halfway mark in this first month. Congratulations! If you are wondering how your body is doing with removing all the toxins and eliminating candida, make sure to check out the next chapter.

Day 15:

Keto-Friendly Snacks

Yes! Snacks!

Keto snacks are totally doable. In my life as a mom and in my career, I travel a lot. I have been to 41 countries, and have spent a lot of time speaking at conferences and wellness centers. I have an active life and do not always have the time to prepare healthy meals, so I like to keep healthy snacks on hand that will support my body.

There are actually some convenience foods that are Keto-friendly. Protein bars that are especially high in protein are an okay choice. I also like granola or fiber bars. When you are looking at those, RE-Member to do your carb math to determine your net carbs. The higher the fiber, the better. Almonds are healthy and convenient, and they will make you feel full. Meat is a great choice for a Keto lifestyle, but I do not mean jerky or Slim Jims. Those are okay in a pinch, but they are full of nitrates, which are terrible for you. Cacao nibs are really good for you and delicious; I like to throw them in with a bag of almonds for a really filling snack with a ton of vitamins.

Of course, your healthiest low-carb snacks are going to be vegetables. Green veggies, like asparagus, avocado, broccoli, lettuce, spinach, olives, cucumbers, zucchini, and kale are particularly low-carb and high in nutrients. Peppers are also low-carb and the darker the peppers, the more nutrients they have. You can cut up some vegetables and bring them to work or on a plane, but you probably do not want them sitting in your bag for too long, so just be mindful and carry an ice pack or store them in a refrigerator.

The "Vegetarian Vegetable Broth and Seasoning" from Seitenbacher is a broth that I enjoy at the Wellness Centers with which I have worked. It's easy to bring the small can to work and easily mixes with hot water. It is low calorie, zero carbs, and you can get it on Amazon. I love it, especially when it is cold outside. This brand in particular is a good choice, because many of the other brands have sugar and preservatives that make them high in carbs and less nutritious. Also, this brand travels very well. You can throw it in your bag, in your suitcase, in your car, or wherever, and it makes a great instant broth.

Here is a quick list of some more Keto-friendly snacks:

Hardboiled egg
Pork rinds
String cheese
Dark chocolate
Sunflowers seeds
Pumpkin seeds
Fat bombs
Keto smoothie
Lettuce wrap
Flaxseed crackers
Keto chips (I love Quest's
    version)
Moon cheese
Tuna salad
Canned sardines
Keto peanut butter with
    celery sticks
Keto pigs in a blanket

Zucchini chips
Seaweed
Chia seed pudding
Deli meat tray
Sugar-free Jell-O
Olives
Kale chips
Coconut butter
Halo Top ice cream
Keto chocolate pudding (made
    with avocado and
        cacao)
Bacon
Spinach artichoke dip
Keto bark (Choc Zero)
Leafy Greens
Cucumbers
Radishes

Celery   Tomatoes
Olives

Lastly, I encourage you to look at the benefits of Slique™ gum—there are more than I can count, and even more than I am allowed to say, but do your due diligence and look up Slique™ gum, coriander, dill, cinnamon bark, peppermint, ocotea, and bergamot oils; they are helpful for supporting healthy body systems. If you have not been to my YouTube channel, go check it out because there are so many videos that can help support you along the way.

I have more information on this, including specific links, in my Keto Membership www.swiftfire.org/onlineclasses or check out my resources page for more information.

Next up, I will be discussing Keto-friendly drinks that are under 3 carbs!

Day 16:

Keto Drinks Under 3 Carbs

My first recommendation is, of course, to drink a lot of *__water__*. Water is always the best choice, but it is especially crucial while your body is in Ketosis because it helps flush out the toxins.

There are also some non-coffee options. Dandelion blend tea is a great coffee substitute if you are quitting caffeine, and is supportive of your liver health. Slique® tea is good for your healthy body system. Runa is a plant-based energy drink that has only one carb in the entire bottle. Apple cider vinegar is also good for your body and comes in a many different flavors. It is important to keep in mind that there are a lot of carbs in some of those flavored variations, so it would be better to just take a shot of the vinegar or mix it with water. Braggs Limeaid Apple Cider Vinegar has *zero* carbs, so that would be a really good choice for your body. Yerbae is a sparkling water blend that has several flavors and zero carbs. Personally, I love Kevita, which is a store-bought kombucha drink. I have to be careful with those though, because only the lemon-cayenne and hibiscus-cherry flavors are low-carb.

Now we need to look at some protein powders. There is also Garden of Life's Raw Protein and Greens, which you can get at Whole Foods. It has 5 carbs, but there are 3 grams of fiber, making it only 2 net carbs. Even better: it is gluten-free, vegan, raw, dairy-free, and soy-free, and it is made from spinach, kale, broccoli, and alfalfa grass juice, it is organic, has 20 grams of protein, and tastes great. High Performance Nutrition's Protein Zero has about 2 grams of carbs and 20 grams of protein for one scoop. I would use this not as a drink, but as a meal replacement if you are choosing to do intermittent fasting. Slique® Essence is an essential oil and it is delicious, with a minty, refreshing taste—just add a drop or two to water, and be sure to use a glass water container.

We should revisit **water** one more time. Many people struggle with getting enough water throughout the day, but there are a lot of ways to trick yourself into drinking more water. You can drink sparkling water, which comes in a lot of different flavors. These days there are many sparkling water options such as Bubly, Perrier, Spindrift, La Croix, and Polar. San Pellegrino is a mineral sparkling water and it has the highest mineral count out of all the mineral waters I have found. You can also drink club soda if that is your thing. If you are not a fan of sparkling water, there are flavored flat waters such as Hint that have zero carbs, or you can grab the zero-carb water additives. (I have more info on these in my Keto Membership[e] as well.)

Again, please drink a lot of water; it will only do good things for your body. However, if you are a coffee drinker, I have some tips for how to navigate Starbucks in the next chapter.

---

e   Class information can be found at www.swiftfire.org/onlineclasses

Day 17:

Starbucks Hacks

Once you know what you are doing, this will get easier. You CAN enjoy all of your favorite places with a few hacks. I know how popular and fun Starbucks can be, and if you choose to treat yourself AND stay in Ketosis, here are some easy Keto-friendly recipes. Side note: Several of these were introduced to me by my friend, Anna Fogg (thanks, Anna). Several of these ideas also came from our membership group. If you join our interactive group, we have a variety of ideas there daily as we like to experiment with fun and accountability.

- ALWAYS have heavy whipping cream. Ask for it! Add Protein Powder, as each scoop has 1 gram of carbs and 1 gram of fiber, which equal zero net carbs. Use that to make your own custom "meal in a cup" when blended with ice and espresso.

- This tastes like ice cream! Ask for: Venti Passion Tango unsweetened iced tea with one pump of sugar-free vanilla and a big splash of heavy whipping cream, with NO classic, shaken (only 2 carbs).

- Iced Venti Latte, with a big splash of heavy whipping cream and two pumps of sugar-free vanilla (3 carbs).

- Americano with a splash of heavy whipping cream (add Stevia if you require it).

- Americano with a shot of heavy whipping cream and sugar-free cinnamon dolce syrup.

- Shot of espresso (or regular coffee) with heavy whipping cream in place of milk and add a pump or two of sugar-free cinnamon dolce.

- Flat white with a splash of almond milk or heavy whipping cream.

- Iced Doppio Blonde Espresso over ice in a tall cup, with one packet of Stevia/Monk Fruit sweetener and heavy whipping cream.

- Unsweetened, iced green tea with heavy whipping cream.

- Iced green tea, shaken (no carbs).

- Four shots of blonde roast over ice, with one pump of sugar-free vanilla, one pump of sugar-free dolce, and a splash of heavy whipping cream (no classic base).

- Keto Frappuccino: Ask for a coffee frap, substituting half heavy whipping cream and half water for the skim milk (no classic base).

- Hot tea without sugar (unless you do Stevia).

- Basic coffee: Ask for any coffee with any flavor sugar-free syrup (or not), and leave room for heavy whipping cream. RE-Member, sugar-free syrup is just an option, not a necessity.

- Bulletproof coffee: Ask for any coffee but leave extra room and ask for 4 tablespoons of grass-fed butter (such as KerryGold, which they carry) and a child's cup of heavy whipping cream on the side.

Starbucks has some Keto food choices as well, such as moon cheese or string cheese. Some stores have the Creminelli salami and cheese tray, which has zero carbs. I usually grab 2-3 when I go for snacks or a meal later. Lots of great choices!

I included this chapter because I want to show you how easy it can be to incorporate the Keto lifestyle into *your* life. The next chapter is about conscious language, which is a mindset that will help you so much as you transition into full Keto.

Day 18:

Conscious Language and Divine Health

You are over halfway through the beginning of your Keto journey!

Next up, I want to discuss the importance of CONSCIOUS LANGUAGE during Keto—and during *LIFE*.

There is so much power in what we are saying *over* ourselves and others. There is power in what we are saying *to* ourselves. Science proves that what we say really *matters*. I invite you to read my book, *The Science of Miracles, RE-Membering the Frequency of Love*[f], for more insight on how we can change our lives for the better as we co-create with ease.

God spoke the world into existence. Source just said, "Let there be LIGHT." And there was Light and still is Light. That God is in you, co-creating with you now, with every word you say.

If you have never studied the science of Cymatics, check it out. I also encourage you to look into *Hidden Messages in the Water* by Dr. Emoto. Both of these will give you great insights, and if you go to YouTube, you can have a visual experience as well. It is so fascinating to me, the science connection. What we say has sound and resonance, and this

---

f   A part of this chapter is an excerpt from my book, *The Science of Miracles*. See www.swiftfire.org.

sound/resonance not only has frequency, but it also *creates*. Thoughts matter, feelings matter, and, yep... our *words MATTER*.

I am going to mention a few Bible verses here, but please know that as I mention these scriptures, I am coming at this from a place of quantum physics, not religion or denomination. I am a spirit being and I happen to love God; you may have your version and that is totally cool with me. Your road and path are your own, but seriously, check these out:

"By your words you will be justified and by your words you shall be condemned." (Matthew 12:37)

"Speak those things that are not as though they were." (Romans 4:17)

"There is death and life in the power in the tongue." (Proverbs 18:21)

"He sent out His word and healed them." (Psalm 107:20)

"Whoever would love life and see good days must keep their tongue from evil and their lips from deceitful speech." (1 Peter 3:10)

"Speak with wisdom and faithful instruction is on her tongue." (Proverbs 31:26)

"Set a guard over my mouth, keep watch over my lips." (Psalm 141:3)

"The words of the reckless pierce like swords but the tongue of the wise brings healing." (Proverbs 12:18)

These are just a few of the scriptures that talk about the power of words and language. There is an awesome book on the subject called *Conscious*

Language[g] by my dear friend and co-missioner, Robert Tennyson Stevens[h], that I encourage you to read to gain even more insight.

We know that conscious language, your word choices, and the vibration of your words actually have a major effect on not only yourselves and your health, but also on your environment; a lesson I learned early on.

Words direct and shape energy.

When you use words, you cast your thoughts into the Earth's magnetic force and energy field, which creates reality (for good or bad). Choose wisely.

For example, if you say that you "want to lose weight," the word "want" means "lack," so the energy focus is on keeping you at lack or not having yet. Saying you "want to release weight," Re-Lease....RE means to do again....lease means to pay for something over and over that you do not own." Not an ideal word choice.

A better choice might be, "I enjoy my size 8 jeans" (you fill in the size of your choice), or even, "I enjoy my divine health now!"

These are just a few things in language that shape your life. Again, I invite you to be consciously aware of what you speak out loud and even your *inner* chatter. You matter.

---

g   Available at the swiftfire.org bookstore
h   Robert Tennyson Stevens is the founder and CEO of Mastery Systems Corporation. He is a pioneer in the influence of language, imagination, facilitation, and body language.

Day 19:

The Process and the Journey

On Day 19, I choose to share with you a little more about the process and journey that is Keto. There is a reason why I call Keto a lifestyle: It is about more than just the first 31 days. It is not short-term, nor is it a "quick fix." For me, this has been a lifestyle change. The weight I transmuted, the energy I gained, the Divine Health I am feeling was not an overnight experience.

Sure, some people have awesome experiences where they get on a diet and they transmute 30 pounds in a few weeks or drop a few inches. It was not like that for me; it has taken me several years to lose one hundred pounds. I saw results right away, but then I started to plateau. I kept at it because I was feeling good and noticed that my health was the best it had ever been, and now, a few years later, I can say that I had to change my lifestyle to get to where I am.

I RE-Member the first day I went to the store to buy some new clothes because I had left behind the size 24 items and dropped down to a size 18. I did not even know where to shop because I had been shopping in plus sizes for so long. Then I was a size 16, a size 14, a size 12; the weight just kept coming off and I realized that this was a lifestyle that gave me everything I required to have my own Divine Health. It was not about the weight shifts, it was about *how good I felt in my body and my spirit.*

Important note: do not let a scale or a waist size determine how you feel about yourself. There will be times when you are one weight and there will be times when your sizes change drastically, but this is not a sprint, it is a life marathon. There is no "run and get to the goal." This is a process, and it is *for life*.

Will I ever go back to eating carbs? Probably not. Keto is my life and I will do this forever because there are so many benefits. I no longer have joint pain, I love my body, I am not bloated, I have great energy, clarity in my thoughts and memory AND IT IS GOOD FOR ME TO SAY NO TO SUGAR.

That is my encouragement to you today. Stay the course and know that this is a journey that makes life so amazing. I am proud of you for sticking with it and dedicating yourself to living the best, and healthiest life you can. You should be proud of yourself, too, and excited that you love yourself enough to take care of your health.

Day 20:

Keto Restaurant Hacks

I love to go out to restaurants and honestly I don't particularly love cooking (lol). If my husband and kids are out of town, I go out to eat or honestly I don't eat. My travel schedule, teaching all over the world, also lends more towards eating out. That can seem like a really daunting thing when you are doing Keto, but it is surprisingly easy. The first hack is a plain bunless burger, which you can order at any dine-in restaurant with burgers on the menu. Sometimes they will wrap it in lettuce. I add bacon, cheese, and onions to mine because, as you know, most condiments have loads of sugar and carbs.

If you go somewhere a little more upscale, like a steak house, I recommend ordering a nice steak with some butter or sour cream and a side of vegetables. If you go the salad route, be sure to add some extra meat to it and leave off the croutons. Oil and vinegar make a great, clean dressing, or you can get some packets of Keto-friendly salad dressing such as Tessemae. That brand has several low or zero carb salad dressings that are delicious and available in 1-oz packets. As for soups, aim for broth-based varieties that do not include potatoes or grains.

There is a variety of different types of cuisine available. Maybe you like to go out for Mexican food. I recommend getting fajitas, carnitas, or salad with no tortillas, rice, or beans. It can be hard to find Keto-friendly food at Italian restaurants because most sauces have flour, cream, and even sugar in them—and, of course, pasta is not Keto. You can always ask for unbreaded or plain baked chicken breasts. These days, more pizzerias are coming out with cauliflower crusts and even crustless pizzas, which are basically the cheese, toppings, and sauce baked in a dish. Chinese food is probably the hardest menu to stay within Keto guidelines, so I typically stay away from it. However, hibachi restaurants are usually okay if you stick with meats, vegetables, and garlic with no sauce.

Breakfast restaurants are probably the most Keto-friendly. You can get eggs, bacon, sausage, and vegetables. You have to be careful, though, because some restaurants like IHOP put pancake mix or flour in their scrambled eggs and omelets.

Seafood restaurants are another great option for following the Keto meal plan. Be sure to opt for grilled or boiled seafood, as fried or battered seafood is not going to be healthy.

As for fast food, Popeye's Chicken has something called blackened tenders and naked tenders. You have to ask for them, but there are only a few carbs in each serving so it is worth it to ask. Jimmy Johns does the Unwich, which is basically any of their sandwiches wrapped in lettuce without the bread, which is a great option on the go. Subway does chopped salads, which are good because you can control what goes in them. Again, watch your dressings, because many of them are bad for you, but oil and vinegar are always a good choice. At Chipotle or Taco Bell, you can order a salad bowl. We love Buffalo Wild Wings. We get the traditional wings because they do not have any kind of added breading or anything on them. Your safest bet there is the buffalo sauce, garlic parmesan, or a dry rub.

If bread is a temptation when you go out to dinner, ask them not to bring it to the table. If you are dining with people who are not on Keto or who love bread, ask them to put it on the other side of the table away from you. Do not be afraid to ask for things without sauce. Ask for modifications; a lot of places now have a gluten-free menu that is a good place to start, because those items will not have flour or gluten, and then you can modify from there. Most importantly, know where you are going in advance. That way, you can look up the menu online and figure out what you will order ahead of time based on the nutrition facts and availability.

If restaurants seem doable, but travel still feels impossible, then the next chapter is just for you. I will show you that it is *totally* possible to travel and stay in Ketosis.

Day 21:

Travel Tips

Travel options have changed tremendously over the years. Thank God airports and even gas stations are finally realizing that some people actually want healthy choices when they travel. One of my favorite things to do is travel with my family. I know that there are always a lot of things to prepare before we depart for a trip, and now that I have this Keto lifestyle, snacks and meals are just another thing to prepare. There are a few generic tips that are always helpful. ALWAYS PACK HEALTHY SNACKS WITH YOU!

I like to portion out my snacks so that I know exactly how much of everything I am ingesting. Take macadamia nuts, for example. I love them and they are a great source of healthy fat, but just 10 macadamia nuts have more than 200 calories. So, if I do not portion them out I might end up eating a whole can, which could be a thousand calories or more. I always bring a big bottle of water because it is so important to stay hydrated, especially while traveling. It also makes buying an unhealthy drink at the gas stations less tempting.

As for which snacks to bring, you cannot go wrong with veggies, nuts, boiled eggs, cheese, protein bars, protein chips, or meat. I also like to make some fat bombs and bring them with me. Fat bombs are little Keto-friendly treats made with nut butters, coconut oil, cocoa powder, cream cheese, or avocado. There are a bunch of different ways to make them. Most recipes have zero carbs, and contain a lot of healthy fat and very little sugar. (See my chapter on snacks.)

You can take the restaurant tips from the previous chapter and apply them to hotel breakfasts as well. Be careful with what you order and ask questions. I once ordered eggs at a hotel and they kicked me out of Ketosis. I could not figure out why until the next day, when I peeked behind the preparation door of the hotel. The eggs were from a ***BOX!*** When I asked about them, I learned they were FULL of carbs. Ask for REAL EGGS. Also ask for substitutions, or do your intermittent fasting until you can get somewhere else with healthier choices.

The other thing that I have noticed when I am trying to eat out is that the food is always very salty. That makes you retain fluid, and we do not want that because we want the scales to move and our bodies to change. Another example is, if you are the type of person who likes to get their coffee to go, it is okay to talk to your barista and ask them for help with making the perfect drink.

Most importantly—plan ahead. Everything is easier when you pre-plan your snacks and meals.

In the next few chapters, I will be covering some of the experiences that people have on their Keto journeys.

Day 22:

Medical Reasons for Plateau

One of the things that people often see in the first few weeks of starting Ketogenic living is a drop in the number on the scale. A lot of us pay too much attention to that number on the scale and we think that it tells us the truth, but it does not. That number does not have to change for your health to change for the better.

I want you to think of our fat cells as having different shapes and sizes. In our pre-Keto lifestyle, our glucose-driven diet made our pancreas release insulin, which forced glucose into our cells where it became triglycerides. The cells used what they needed of the glucose, and then they stored the rest. When you went into Ketosis and stopped taking in all that glucose, you began to release those Ketones to use up that fat. As the fat exits the cell, it does not change shape, because it expects your body to yo-yo back to your former diet. Then, that fat cell is the same size and it pulls water in, which means it is still the same weight. So, you will get on the scale and the number will be the same, your measurements will be the same, but your body is still getting healthier even though you cannot see it.

That is the point when a lot of people quit, even though they should keep going. They give up and they bring the glucose back into their diet and those fat cells say, "See? We knew it was smart to keep the same shape because now the glucose is back." So, those people are training their bodies to hold onto those big fat cells. Here is how you will know that the Keto lifestyle is working. First, ignore the scale. Instead, get a shirt or jeans that may be a size too small. Stick with your Keto lifestyle and try the shirt or jeans on at the same time every day. Soon after you plateau, you will start to notice that shirt fitting better.

Other things that can cause plateaus? Hormones, lack of sleep, or too much fake sugar in your diet. Also, some prescription medications, vitamins, and supplements can kick you out of Ketosis and cause a plateau.

Please consider "non-scale" victories are *just as important.* For instance, feeling better, high energy, your body FREE of carbs, cleansed, working and functioning better, better sleep, getting your brain back! Think of these amazing changes in you!

The key is: Do not give up. KEEP GOING and continue reading to get my tips for keeping up that momentum.

Day 23:

Tips for Keeping Up Momentum

You are doing great! You are at the point where you can really feel the effects of the Keto lifestyle. You have lost some weight, your energy is up, and your sleep is amazing. This is also the point when some people start to notice the plateau that I mentioned in the last chapter. Just keep in mind that, even if you feel like nothing is happening, things are definitely still happening.

Allow me to share a few tips to keep you motivated. As I said, do not look at the scale. Do not worry about whether the "diet" is "working." If your sticks say that you are in Ketosis, then it is working. All that matters is how you feel, what you are thinking about, and the clarity in your mind. Just keep doing what you are doing. It has helped and has been beneficial so far, so just keep going and stick with it.

This is not the time to retreat or be discouraged, thinking that things are not moving for you. They are moving, it is just not visible to your eyes because it occurs on a cellular level. Keep going, and do not use this as an excuse to quit or take cheat days. If you do cheat, you are going to get out of Ketosis and have to start all over again, and we do not want that.

Increase your intake of warm lemon water in the morning and at night, because part of the issue could be that you are not releasing and circulating out those toxins. We want to detox the body from any chemicals that could be causing an issue while you are melting the fat, because now they are going to have to go somewhere and they will head straight into your bloodstream. Drink more.

You may also choose to increase your exercise. If you have not added exercise or cardio into your week, definitely consider just doing a 20 to 30 minute walk 3 to 4 times a week. It does not have to be outside, but go to the mall or hop on a treadmill for 20 minutes. You can even just do 20 minutes of jumping jacks in your living room—anything that gets your body moving and your blood circulating to get those toxins out.

Consider intermittent fasting. Sometimes a fast day or a fast period will shock the body into that next level. Every now and then, I will do a fast for an entire day. If you are already doing intermittent fasting, you can bump up your schedule to increase your fast, or you can choose to do a one-day fast. Whatever you choose that is outside of your norm, a fast can be very beneficial to your body.

Lastly, have you considered a liver and gallbladder cleanse? If your liver is on point and functioning, then not only will you produce more Ketones, but you are also going to have better function overall for all the things your liver does for your metabolism, digestion, immunity, heart, and so much more.

If you have not done a cleanse, now is the time. An average 30-year-old who has not done a cleanse yet can have up to 2,000 stones in their liver. That has a major negative impact on the body. If you choose to do a cleanse, make sure you choose one in which you can see the stones exit your body. Otherwise, you are not doing a real cleanse. I have a 4-day guided Cleanse Membership for this[i], just look in the resources section for more information. If you can reset your liver and gallbladder, you can increase your metabolism and energy. I did four cleanses, four

---

i   Class information can be found at www.swiftfire.org/onlineclasses

months in a row until ALL the stones were out. It totally changed the game for me!

You are doing so well in this journey, and you should be very proud of yourself for making a lifestyle change that will improve every area of your life.

Day 24:

Why Is My Stick Trace?

I would like to offer some information for people who are using the Keto sticks and have noticed that they might have been kicked out of Ketosis. Sometimes, when you are more involved and fully in Ketosis, there are seven different reasons why your sticks are still trace and why you may not get the same color you may have had in the beginning.

The number one reason why you may not see color on your sticks yet is because there may be hidden sugar or carbs in your diet. You have to be especially careful when you are going out to eat and really track everything that you ingest, because that will help you determine which foods are kicking you out of Ketosis. Reading labels is so crucial to the Ketosis process. For example, I went to Starbucks to get my "Pink Drink," and when I took a sip, I noticed that it tasted sweeter than normal. When I looked at the label, I saw that they had put regular cream instead of heavy whipping cream in my drink. Well, cream is milk, and there is a lot of sugar in milk, so if I had finished the entire drink I would have been kicked out of Ketosis.

I went to Waffle House the other day and ordered an omelet. I had two bites before I realized I had forgotten to ask whether they were real eggs or if they used milk in their eggs. Even as a "pro" in this Keto journey, I make mistakes and sometimes get kicked out of Ketosis. We have to be really careful, but also very forgiving with ourselves if we do make a mistake. The good news is that, if you are kicked out of Ketosis, it will be much faster to get back into it the second time around.

This is another reason why I really recommend keto sticks. Because if you use them frequently and you know that before breakfast you were "fine", then eat breakfast and test and you suddenly are not in ketosis anymore, you know it was something that happened at breakfast.

If you do not test until night and you are kicked out you have to deduct and "Sherlock Holmes" your way around what happened for the *whole day*. And honestly, you may never know. If you don't know, this could lead to a repeat mistake with the *same* food kicking you out again. Unless you had fasted most the day there can be any number of things in the equation to consider. I love my sticks.

A second reason why you might be getting kicked out of Ketosis is that you are drinking a whole lot of liquids which are diluting your urine. That is a good thing! It might make your stick appear trace, even though you are still in full-on Ketosis, but at least you are really hydrated.

A third culprit is excess caffeine. We all love our black coffee and our bulletproof coffee, but if you have too much caffeine, that can mess with your sticks.

A fourth factor to watch for is artificial sugars: Xylitol, Splenda, sugar alcohols, and so on. We know that sugar is not Keto-friendly, but a lot of the artificial sugars can also kick you out of Ketosis because, for some of us, the liver views those artificial sugars as toxins. That encourages your liver to eliminate the toxins before it creates Ketones, which is not what we want.

The fifth reason is a little tricky. If you are in full-on Ketosis and find yourself with a lot of energy, you might spend that energy exercising or cleaning. If you are doing that, and your body is using the Ketones to break down the fuel, then you are using that fuel to expend your energy. As a result, it may not show up on the sticks because you are actually using it up. If you are feeling great, sleeping well, and being very careful with your eating plan, then you are likely still in Ketosis and you will not have to worry too much. Sometimes excessive protein can be the culprit. I have never had that happen, but I have heard other people who have eaten too much protein and it has impacted their Ketone production.

Stress is yet another reason why your sticks are trace. If you live in a high-stress state with cortisol flowing through your body, that is going to mess with your Ketone production.

Another reason you may not show you're in Ketosis is due to your EXPIRED sticks, so check the expiration date. Whenever I open a new bottle, I immediately mark the lid with a Sharpie because they only last six months from the date you open them. You might also have gotten a bad batch. The only way to know if the sticks are the cause is to test regularly, three or four times a day. Keep the sticks in all your bathrooms, in your purse, in your car; that way you will always have them available.

If your sticks are reading only trace amounts of Ketones despite adhering strictly to plan, it is time to look into your lifestyle to find these hidden culprits. Do not stress if you find out you have been accidentally eating more sugar than you would have liked. Mistakes happen and can be corrected.

Day 25:

Appetite and Keto

I am going to dive into managing your weight and appetite, and how we can help support the body naturally for complete divine health.

Specifically, there are two hormones that we can help modulate, so that our endocrine system is working with us. First is ghrelin, which I like to think of as "growlin'" because it makes you feel hungry and makes your stomach growl. The other hormone is cholecystokinin (CCK), which causes you to feel full. One hormone tells your body to eat, the other tells your body to stop eating.

Most people are not eating quality, nutrient-packed foods. Why is that an issue? Well, CCK is released about 15 minutes after nutrients enter your body. But if you are not eating nutrient-dense foods, then you are just getting a lot of calories and sugar without the nutrition, which means your body will not release the CCK. Your brain thinks that it is still hungry because, even though you have eaten, you have not taken in any nutrients. When eating Keto, we do not count calories, because we are more concerned about nutrients. If you are giving the body the nutrients it needs in healthy, nutritious food instead of carbohydrate- and sugar-packed foods, then you can eat more calories because your body is using the food you are giving it.

When you have Ketones in your body that go into the bloodstream, they modulate the endocrine system. Ketosis helps modulate your endocrine system and CCK, which will help you feel more satiated. Before people try Keto or intermittent fasting, they worry that they will not like it or that they will feel like they are depriving themselves of something. But once people start Keto, they realize that they feel so good about their body and so satisfied that they sometimes *forget to eat.*

I'm not kidding.

Don't believe me? Check out some of the incredible testimonies at the end of the book. Or check out our group FULL of these type situations. Food becomes a faint thought.

Why? On a science level, once you have initially detoxed, you *may* have felt hungry. As your Ketones get in the bloodstream and start turning off the hunger switches, in most cases *you will not feel hungry anymore.* Ketones are an appetite suppressant, so they suppress ghrelin. You will consistently feel full and satisfied in this lifestyle, in addition to having the energy and mental clarity.

Once you are in Ketosis, it is like a light bulb comes on. You feel awake, you feel alive, and you are burning your fat as fuel.

Day 26:

Tips to Maintain Your Ideal Weight

A lot of things contribute to being overweight. Your body runs on fuel and energy because it is a machine. We have 30 to 40 trillion cells in the body, and all these little cells need nutrients and water. So, how can we manage our weight?

1. When your brain knows that it is time to fuel up, it sends messages throughout the body that say, "Hey, let's fuel up." Meaning... "I need nutrients." The problem is that we may not be actually giving the body nutrients. Instead, we may be "fueling up" with junk "food" or processed "food" containing absolutely no nutritional value. If you give yourself real food enriched with vitamins, minerals and thriving life, your body will shut off the hunger message and you stop "feeling" hungry.

2. Your body cannot tell you that it is full until about 30 minutes into eating. If you sit down and devour everything in 10 minutes, you may still feel hungry, so you keep eating. But what really happened was that you did not give your body and your brain time to realize that you are full.

3. Focus on foods that are raw and organic, and stay away from foods with excess sugar.

4. Do not drink water while you are eating. Drink water before you eat and after you eat, not during.

5. Take a few minutes each week to really plan your food. If you can, plan out your meal schedule for the week and then prepare your meals ahead of time.

6. Do not go to the grocery store hungry because you are going to buy everything. That will really help you stay away from relying on prepackaged food.

7. Statistics say that families who eat meals together have children who grow up healthier and with stronger marriages, so try to eat together as a family.

I hope these easy ideas create lasting changes that can help you maintain your ideal body and weight. You may have noticed that "develop good sleeping habits"—a common and crucial weight management tip—is not on this list. That is because sleep is so important to the healthy-weight formula that I have devoted the entire next chapter to it.

Day 27:

What's Sleep Got to Do with It?

Sleep is a **BIG** deal. There is a lot of science and research on the subject, and it all says that sleep is important, especially in maintaining a healthy balance to your body weight. You should have at least 7 to 8 hours of sleep each night. In fact, some studies show that one night's sleep deprivation caused an alarming decrease in insulin sensitivity. You can be on a high-fat diet for six months and it only decreases the sensitivity to 21%, but if you miss just one night of sleep, it decreases insulin sensitivity to 33%. This means your body has a difficult time with insulin, and if you have insulin resistance, then there is an issue with getting rid of high blood sugars.

The time you sleep is as important as the time when you eat. The ideal time when your body releases the most HGH (human growth hormone) is between the hours of 10p.m. to 12 a.m. Dr. Gary Young[j] always said if we sleep during this time period especially, we release more HGH, and it is comparable to four hours of sleep instead of two! So this is key. Are you asleep by then?

I also recommend that you do not eat past 7 p.m. If you go to bed on a full stomach, your body makes a choice to digest or repair, and as

---

j   D. Gary Young (1949-2018) was the founder of Young Living Essential Oils and is known around the world as the father of the modern-day essential oils movement.

mentioned in a previous chapter, digest wins over repair every time. This affects the immunity and the regeneration/balance of the body.

It is more important that your sleep helps to balance your body, maintain immunity, and restore whatever needs your body's attention at that time. Do whatever you can to eat an earlier dinner and make it *light*.

Day 28:

Documentaries to Further Your Learning

Here are a few documentaries on sugar and food that I encourage you to watch to help you _reprogram_. These will help you understand the reasoning behind the Keto lifestyle and how much better it is for your body. I find that if you understand _why_ you are doing this you have better success. You can find them on Netflix and Amazon.

1. THAT SUGAR FILM
   Damon Gameau embarks on a unique experiment to document the effects of a high-sugar diet on a healthy body, consuming only foods that are commonly perceived as "healthy." Through this entertaining and informative journey, Damon highlights some of the issues that plague the sugar industry, and where sugar lurks on supermarket shelves. That Sugar Film will forever change the way you think about "healthy" food.

2. FED UP
   This is the movie the food industry does not want you to see. Fed Up blows the lid off everything we thought we knew about food and weight loss, revealing a 30-year campaign by the food industry, aided by the U.S. Government, to mislead and confuse the American public, resulting in one of the largest health epidemics in history. From Katie Couric, Laurie David (Oscar winning producer

of <u>An Inconvenient Truth</u>), and director Stephanie Soechtig, <u>Fed Up</u> will change the way you eat forever.

3. FAT, SICK, AND NEARLY DEAD

Overweight, loaded up on steroids and suffering from a debilitating autoimmune disease, Joe Cross was at the end of his rope and the end of his hope. With doctors and conventional medicine unable to help, Joe traded in junk food and hit the road with a juicer and generator in tow, vowing only to drink fresh fruit and vegetable juice for 60 days. Across 3,000 miles Joe had one goal in mind: To get off his pills and achieve a balanced lifestyle.

4. FOOD, INC.

Documentary filmmaker, Robert Kenner, examines how mammoth corporations have taken over all aspects of the food chain in the United States, from the farms where our food is grown to the chain restaurants and supermarkets where it is sold. Narrated by author and activist Eric Schlosser, the film features interviews with average Americans about their dietary habits, commentary from food experts like Michael Pollan, and unsettling footage shot inside large-scale animal processing plants.

5. SUPER SIZE ME

While examining the influence of the fast food industry, Morgan Spurlock personally explores the consequences on his health from a diet of solely McDonald's food for one month.

6. SUGAR COATED

This documentary investigates the history of the food industry's use of sugar, its health impact on society, and the politics of the "new tobacco."

7. FOOD MATTERS

"Let thy Food be thy Medicine and thy Medicine be thy Food."
— Hippocrates

That is the message from the founding father of modern medicine echoed in the controversial new documentary film, Food Matters, from first-time Producer-Directors James Colquhoun and Laurentine ten Bosch.

"With nutritionally-depleted foods, chemical additives, and our tendency to rely upon pharmaceutical drugs to treat what is wrong with our malnourished bodies, it is no wonder that modern society is getting sicker. Food Matters sets about uncovering the trillion dollar worldwide "Sickness Industry" and giving people some scientifically verifiable solutions for curing disease naturally." – James Colquhoun

And in what promises to be the most contentious idea put forward, the filmmakers have interviewed several world leaders in nutrition and natural healing who claim that not only are we harming our bodies with improper nutrition, but also that the right kind of foods, supplements, and detoxification can be used to treat chronic illnesses as fatal as terminally-diagnosed cancer.

8. HUNGRY FOR CHANGE
    From the creators of the best-selling documentary Food Matters® comes another hard-hitting film certain to change everything you thought you knew about food and nutrition. Hungry for Change exposes shocking secrets the diet, weight loss, and food industries do not want you to know about deceptive strategies designed to keep you coming back for more. Find out what is keeping you from having the body and health you deserve and how to escape the diet trap forever.

Day 29:

Crystals

Do not freak out on me, I promise you I am not getting whoo whoo on you! There is actually a science to this. If you would have told me a few years ago that I would be writing a chapter on crystals, I would have laughed at you just like some of you may be laughing at me right now. But, crystals **do** work. There is a science to it, and for those who believe in the Bible, they are actually biblical.

Crystals are a structured form, and though the stones themselves are not magic, they do carry a vibration and a code specific to their form. That vibration is transferable, and whether you are one of the people who feel it or not, the vibration still exists. Crystals form only in the right circumstances, based on high temperatures, gasses, and the earth's crust. As they cool, the constituent atoms arrange themselves into a more stable relationship. This creates a three-dimensional repeating pattern as the crystal lattices into a shape in which every atom has found the most stable balance arrangement possible.

Even if crystals are exposed to chaos, they have the ability to keep their structure, because they are so stable. Think about that. We may be in an environment of chaos, or we may be in a chaotic state, but we can add something stable to our bio field, our body, or (more specifically) on our skin to create a calming effect. Each individual crystal offers its own unique vibration and support to us. There is a huge range of different crystals, minerals, and gemstones that are all God-given to encourage us to reach our best, higher self. They bring a sense of order and balance, not just physically and emotionally, and are effective for mental health. I have interviewed several experts and have learned that there are specific crystals that can help with addiction and stress management.

I will give you my own personal testimony. Previously, I mentioned that I like to wear hematite. My father was in the military, so we traveled quite a lot. I spent a few years in Europe when I was growing up. Over there, it is common to drink alcohol. The pubs are open for children, McDonald's sells beer, and wine is just a normal part of everyday life. People in Europe do not drink in excess the way they sometimes do in the US. When we came back to the States, it became a normal practice for me to have a glass of wine with dinner as an adult. (With the Keto lifestyle, I usually choose a red wine because it is lower in carbs.)

I was looking for energetic help in all things, and I landed in a crystal shop. For some reason, I found that I was really drawn to hematite and amethyst, so I bought both that day. I put the amethyst next to my bed because I heard it helps with sleep, and I bought a hematite bracelet for my right wrist. That night, I tasted my wine at dinner and it was disgusting. It tasted like metal! I asked my husband, "What in the world are we drinking?" He informed me that we were drinking my favorite bottle of wine. I absolutely could not believe him. I even walked to the kitchen and opened the refrigerator to see for myself what we were drinking. Lo and behold, it was truly my favorite bottle of wine. I thought I must be mistaken; that there must be something wrong with this bottle. Maybe it is a bad batch? Is that even possible?

So, the next day, I got a new bottle and the same thing happened. The wine tasted disgusting. I continued with this several times until I finally gave up. For some reason, my taste buds had changed. About a week later, I was working on a highlighted crystal in my crystal membership group. I chose hematite as the highlight for the week. I had absolutely no knowledge regarding hematite up to that point, so I started researching. I saw that the number one thing that hematite is good for is breaking addictions and reprogramming your brain!

I could not even believe that there was such a thing, to be honest.

So, I searched the words "crystals" and "addictions" to see what came up. *Hematite and amethyst!*

I quickly did the math and realized that my change of taste buds happened the same day I put the amethyst next to my bedside table and wore the hematite bracelet.

I never saw myself as an addict when it came to wine. I never drank in excess, although I did enjoy a glass of wine at dinner, particularly with certain foods. Yet, there I was, unable to drink wine anymore, and I have not had it since.

The crystal changed the vibration in my body to not be able to receive the lower vibration of wine. Since then, I have done further studies on how crystals can help in all areas of our lives. If this is a topic of interest for you, I really do hope that you will join me in my members-only *Crystal, Oils, Science and the Bible* group because you could benefit immensely from the discussions and topics.

Below is a compiled, personal list of specific crystals and stones that have helped me and many others, and may help you, too.

Top Crystals for Addictions
- Hematite
- Amethyst
- Carnelian
- Clear quartz
- Tiger eye
- Rose quartz
- Citrine

- Black Obsidian
- Howlite
- Amber

For more education on crystals, I have published some Crystal, Oils, and Decree cards available on my website book store (www.swiftfire. org). They are one of a kind flash cards that include crystals, their support to us, decrees and companion oils. Trust me, check them out!

I also have my *Crystals, Oils, Science and the Bible* class and membership you can go to www.swiftfire.org/onlineclasses. This is a one year membership full of classes, videos, posts, testimonies and tips on the subject. You will love it!

And if you are still with me after an entire chapter on how crystals can support your Keto journey, then keep reading. I developed an entire chapter just for you, about which oils and supplements can also support you.

Day 30:

Oils, Supplements, and Research to Support Your Journey

For your journey with essential oils, I hand-selected some of my personal favorite oils and supplements that have helped support my healthy body systems. There are thousands of others, so please do your due diligence in researching why they are helpful and how they can help you personally. You may not require any of these but I have seen them help in my own life as well as my clients' lives.

Supplements

- Probiotics Life 9™
- Essentialzyme™
- OmegaGize™
- Super B™
- Super C™
- Mineral supplements
- MultiGreens™
- Slique Tea™
- Immupro™
- Sleep Essence™
- ComforTone™
- Parafree™

Essential Oils

- Ocotea
- Lemon
- Lime
- Orange
- Frankincense
- Sacred Frankincense™
- Citrus Fresh™
- Bergamot
- Digize™
- Valor ™
- Valerian
- Motivation™
- Into the Future™
- Envision™
- Transformation™
- Believe™
- En-R-Gee™
- Roman chamomile
- Coriander
- Nutmeg
- Endoflex™
- Progessence Plus™
- Spearmint
- Peppermint
- Juva Flex™
- Juva Cleanse™
- Juva Tone™
- Juvapower™
- Ledum

Day 31:

Conclusion

You did it! You made it 31 days into the Keto journey. I am so proud of you for choosing your Divine Health over and over again, every day with each and every decision you make about what you choose to put into your body. I want you to take some time to really check in with your body. How are you feeling? What improvements have been made in your life? Are you sleeping better? Feeling more energetic? Are you experiencing better clarity?

<u>I would love to hear your testimonies! So keep me posted!</u>

You can find me on social media **@drsharnael**. DM me!

I invite you to continue living this lifestyle as I have because it is an amazing feeling! Do you agree?

RE-Member, this is all about so much more than the number on the scale. It really is about treating your body with the love and respect it deserves. That means feeding it with nutrient-dense foods that allow your body to perform efficiently and effectively. It means getting enough sleep, drinking enough water, exercising and fasting as necessary.

Listen to your body, it will tell you when it is full; it will tell you when it needs rest. Honor those needs, and allow your body to be the best, most whole-self it has ever been.

If you choose to continue on this journey, you are saying YES to a new way of living. You are opening up your life to feeling better than you have ever felt before. It is a lifestyle that requires vigilance and discipline, but the rewards are worth it all!

I am here to support you in your Keto journey and lifestyle. In the next section, you will find a list of resources that you can use to connect with others, learn more about healthy living and Ketosis, and find the support you need as you continue on your journey.

Congratulations! Welcome to your best, most Divine Self.

Xoxo, Dr. Sharnael

Testimonies

I would like to start this chapter with a grateful heart. I have worked with really wonderful clients in this Keto journey and they have allowed me to see just how much starting Keto has improved their lives. I run a few Facebook groups that are filled with incredible, beautiful, supportive people. It is amazing to watch them get off their medications, have higher energy that they can use to play with their children or wake up without alarms, and have the clarity they desire in their lives. Here are a few testimonies from some of my clients that have gone through the Keto Reset 31 Days to New Life membership group.

Dr. Sharnael

* * *

I have always loved food, but it was not until October 2017 that I started to reevaluate my weight. I tried numerous diet plans, including the 21-day challenge and workouts, but nothing really changed. Then, in January 2018, I decided to take part in a Keto group that was being hosted by Dr. Sharnael. The insight and inspiration I received helped set me on a new and exciting path. After three months of being on Keto, I realized that my addiction to food was gone. In the past, if I forgot food that was part of my breakfast or lunch at home, my entire day would be ruined. I would yell, holler, and scream—what some might call "a meltdown." The day I realized the change in myself, I had forgotten an item of food at home. I called my husband, who was waiting for me to show my typical self. He was shocked that I did not have my usual meltdown. A few days later, the situation occurred again. Again, I did not overreact. At that moment I realized that I had been a food addict. Later, my husband confirmed my suspicion.

Today, I am no longer addicted to food. I am 60 pounds lighter and still on the journey to my best health. While not all days are perfect, food no longer has control of me. In her group, Dr. Sharnael has built a community of support and like-minded people. Thank you, Dr. Sharnael, for providing a path of encouragement on my journey to a healthier me.

Lisa McCorkle

* * *

Little did I know that January 3, 2018 would be a life changer for me. I joined Dr. Sharnael's Keto Bootcamp knowing absolutely nothing about Keto. My interest was stirred immediately when I read her post about what sugar does to our body (it is poison). I was a size 10 and never felt I was overweight, but I was plagued with severe back and joint pain, my brain was foggy, and my energy level was very low. What happened within a few weeks seemed magical... my back and joint pain vanished, my energy level soared, and I had clarity of mind! Inches melted away and before I knew it I was a size 4! I can assure you that this Keto Bootcamp from day one has provided my Keto Journey with valuable information, lots of recipes, Keto hacks, and loving support from the members who cheer each other on! My heart's desire is for everyone to experience what I have. Your health is more valuable than gold.

Teresa Wages

* * *

I have lost 12 pounds in one month. Having group support and sharing recipes, ideas, and the support really helps. Sharing the journey with a supportive group that is cheering for my victory is the best! Thank you for doing this!

Michelle Hanson

* * *

I just want to share how far I have come in my life's journey. This is my second challenge since October. I am 58 years of age and have struggled with weight since my early twenties. I tried every diet you could possibly think of and always gained it back with more added. I basically gave up and was surrendering to being overweight. I am very blessed and amazed at what the Lord has done in my life. For over 30 years, I have longed to be thin once again. With constant failures to accomplish this deep down desire, I had really given up. However, HE did not give up. Through a journey into the essential oil lifestyle, I met Dr. Sharnael and she emphasizes how important our bodies (His temples) are to Him. Once I made that connection, my focus became on the health aspect of my life.

Dr. Sharnael Wolverton Sehon introduced me to the Ketogenic lifestyle. With the help and support of Dr. Sharnael and her facebook group, I was able to see dreams come true. Through Keto I am completely prescription free! I have been healed of diabetes, high blood pressure, high cholesterol and I am now in better physical, mental, and spiritual condition than I could have ever asked for.

Since I joined the first challenge, learned and researched Keto. I managed to lose 25 lbs in 21 days. This challenge, so far I have lost an additional 10 pounds, making a total of 35 pounds gone since October.

I have never felt better. I have energy like I am 20 years younger, I actually enjoy yoga exercise; mental clarity allows me to comprehend better and stay focused; and a positive healthy mental attitude allows me to be free of depression. I feel good about myself!

I have two posts on my vision board which say: "my body is a temple, I will not treat it as a trash can" and "the best most underutilized anti-depressant is EXERCISE". This means a lot to motivate me to see how important it is to take care of the temple that HE has entrusted to me, for me to take care of it. Feeding it poison (sugar) benefits no one. I now look forward to each and every day and know that He is with me always. I am truly blessed!

I CHOOSE to be sugar-free! I CHOOSE to be what God intended for me to be physically, mentally, and spiritually, to my fullest ability, which can only be accomplished without feeding my body poison. Lord, I choose this as my new lifestyle and my prayer is for You to give me the strength to always keep you first and resist temptation. I give God all the honor and praise for helping and guiding me to really come to appreciate His temple as a temple and for using Dr. Sharnael to educate me on the body.

My prayer for all of you is for you to never give up; stay strong and He will help you too. Thank you again Dr. Sharnael Wolverton Sehon for being obedient and giving all of us of your time and knowledge.

Renee Jones

* * *

I have made this Keto stuff a lifestyle and choose to do the next Keto Challenge with you. Thank you for instilling a healthy life in me. Yes, I am awake and cleaning at 2 a.m. thanks to my abundant energy.

Sheila Wilson

* * *

This group is amazing. The support is fabulous. I just want to share some of my and my husband's results. I am down 45 pounds and 3 sizes. My husband is within 5 pounds of his high school weight and has gone from 2 insulin shots of 22 units each to no shots some days and only 1 of 22 units on others. It is the first time in 20 years he has been able to lose. We are so blessed to have joined and have the support of Dr. Sharnael Wolverton Sehon.

Alma Walker

* * *

I have lost a total of 6 lbs and 11 inches! Woop! Woop! My energy and clarity are great! My bloat is down! Thank you Dr. Sharnael Wolverton Sehon for believing and teaching us!

Jessica Sera Schultz

* * *

I've been on the Keto wagon since October and it's been part of a huge shift in my life. At the end of January, I'd gotten into my smallest size pants ever. The past few weeks I've noticed they've been looser too. I just went into a store to find a couple new pair and I now fit into a size 14. This is huge for me! I may have been 14 when I last wore that size!

Sarah Blair

* * *

Before, I was lethargic; no motivation, I did not want to get out of bed. I have a lot of floor to sweep, and I could not mop and sweep in one day, I had to choose one or the other because doing just one had me on my back for a couple days. This past weekend, I pressure washed outside, from the back door all the way around to the front door (and I have a big driveway), and I was fine. I was a little sore, but not lying in bed in pain like I would have been. It was exciting! Before, I hurt all the time. All my joints were always hurting. Now, I have not had any problems! I wake up and go, and I have to make myself go to sleep at night. I have been doing the intermittent fasting and I set the goal of fasting until lunchtime every day, but I always go past that to at least one or two o'clock. I am still learning what I need to eat, but it is easier now. I never calculated exactly how much I lost in inches although I transmuted 14 pounds, but I am trying not to focus on that, which is important! I want to get smaller but, with previous diets, I would focus too much on the scale. This time, all of my focus has been on my sticks. If I go below that middle color then I start to worry. The sticks have been super motivating and I use them all the time.

Jvona Jambon

* * *

My big thing was finding a picture of me and my husband from 1994, and seeing how healthy we were and how much we just let ourselves go. I was addicted to sugar since I was a child because of trauma, so it has been a big thing for me to get that monkey off my back. The third reason I got into Keto was that, back in 2008, we started dieting. Then we both fell off the bandwagon and the first thing I noticed was the energy issue, I was staying in bed and did not want to get up. If I did get up, I went straight to the gym, but I would pump myself with a bunch of energy stuff so I could do what I needed to do. I had that brain fog and my confidence was not there. Now, I have signed up for so many classes because I have had such clarity and confidence. But boy, the energy was off the charts, and the clarity. I did not even trust myself doing classes because I would forget so much stuff and the fog was just there, so now I have the confidence to do that. That was a big thing for me. I have scheduled a couple classes and some one-on-ones, because I have more confidence to do it. I have been yo-yo dieting since forever, but when I started Keto, I lost 15.6 pounds in 21 days! I realize that a lot of it was water, but that is cool! I use those Keto sticks every time I go. The other thing I want to encourage everyone to do is to really heed Dr. Sharnael's advice. Like, when she says to cut the Keto sticks in half and put them everywhere. Do that! She does not give that advice for no reason, so listen to everything she is saying because it has kept me on track.

Jeannie Ellis

* * *

We started our Keto journey in January of 2018. Over the course of a year and a half, Gene lost 60 pounds and Teri lost 45 pounds. There were lots of ups and downs, but once we figured out what our macros were and started tracking, it became easier. We could not have done this if it were not for the education, inspiration, and challenges from Dr. Sharnael. She made it fun and interesting to keep going, even when it seemed too tough. We cannot tell you how much we appreciate all of her help. We both feel great and more energetic, but the best part is that Gene was able to come off of his blood pressure medicine, which he had been on for over 20 years. We continue to keep the Keto way of life. We enjoy the foods we eat and have fun making new recipes.

Gene and Teri Backlund

* * *

I just wanted to thank you for everything you've done for the Keto Challenge! I went into the challenge wanting to lose a few pounds, but more than anything, wanting to understand how to eat healthier in my everyday life. My husband and I both lost about 10 pounds each, and we have been loving the healthy meals! I feel like I have a much better understanding of healthy foods, & I love not being addicted to sugar & processed foods. Thank you for all the teaching videos & the encouragement! The way you have used your influence with friends & in YL to help change people's lives is inspiring!

Jessica Boone

* * *

I started this new way of life January 1, 2018. *Now*, over 70 pounds and 57+ inches transmuted. By the grace of God with every layer of fat transmuted there has been mental, emotional and spiritual breakthrough from lies I had believed: I wasn't enough, wasn't beautiful enough, talented enough, enough for someone to marry, the list could go on. Through tears and joyous victory I am still on my journey canceling and clearing all the lies and replacing them with the truth of who I am. I am Divine Health, I am His, I am Beautiful, I am worth it, I am love and I am more than enough, through Him I am perfect. My heart is so full of gratitude for Dr. Sharnael Wolverton Sehon, thank you for being Light, Life and Love to all God places in your sphere of influence. Much love Dr. Sharnael, may God truly bless you beyond measure.

Amanda Coberley Blair

* * *

I wanted to thank you for the prize. I have met a big goal: down 50 lbs in a year. Through your journey I was able to reset and clear a lot of "weight" I was carrying. I am so blessed to be a part of your team. I look forward to having your team with me as I complete my goal of another 70 lbs transmuted!

Elaina Malcolm

* * *

Praise! In 20 days I have chosen to say goodbye or transmuted 10lbs and I'm down 15 inches. I never thought I would ever go down in lbs. But the best thing is I'm so happy and energized. Sleep could be better, but I know this sleep is temporary because my 1yr old daughter has 7 teeth coming in. I choose victory!

Samantha M. Schroll

* * *

18 pounds transmuted, but much more than weight, inches have melted from my body! Scales do not measure inches lost, clarity of mind, inflammation vanishing, or energy! As you RE-Member this, your Keto journey is about everything I have mentioned because I am living proof! There are no words large enough to express my love for Dr. Sharnael and just what she has meant to my life. When I think about her and the

tremendous light that shines in her, through her—my eyes fill with tears of joy. What a difference she has made in the lives of so many! I share my story with everyone. It is my heart's desire for all to take this journey with me and to live abundantly.

Teresa Wages

* * *

This is the 4th time I have done keto but this is the first time, because of your mentoring and the support of others, that I have been successful in transmuting weight and size. Usually I have felt so sick that I have given up! I am sleeping better, or should I say waking up better, and feeling ALIVE both mentally, emotionally, spiritually and physically for the first time in YEARS. I have not had to rely on my B12 shots to get me through the week. My digestion is better and my energy levels have improved. My skin is less dry and I know my adrenals and thyroid are happier. I'm a Nurse and a Naturopath and I know the knowledge I have gained (and continue to learn) will go on to help others too. Thank you so much for the leadership and you have given to us to change our worlds. Much love.

Donna Maree

* * *

I LOVE getting these testimonies and look forward to hearing yours!! I think it is really important for all of us to put voice to what we're feeling and what we're going through, to where this journey actually brought us, and to where we're going. Please report your journey to me @drsharnael. It is really important that you allow this lifestyle to reprogram your body while you work on reprogramming your mind. Keto is not a binge diet, or a yo-yo diet, or a fad; it is a way of life that is having a tangible, positive impact on the men and women who commit to making the change.

Endnotes

1. Avena, Nicole M et al. "Evidence for sugar addiction: behavioral and neurochemical effects of intermittent, excessive sugar intake." *Neuroscience and biobehavioral reviews* vol. 32,1 (2007): 20-39. doi:10.1016/j.neubiorev.2007.04.019 https://www.healthline.com/health/food-nutrition/experts-is-sugar-addictive-drug

2. Cronise, Raymond J et al. "The "metabolic winter" hypothesis: a cause of the current epidemics of obesity and cardiometabolic disease." *Metabolic syndrome and related disorders* vol. 12,7 (2014): 355-61. doi:10.1089/met.2014.0027

3. https://www.johnshopkinshealthreview.com/issues/spring-summer-2016/articles/understanding-inflammation

4. https://bangordailynews.com/2013/04/04/health/how-carbs-are-throwing-your-hormones-out-of-whack/

5. https://amazingdiscoveries.org/AD-Magazine-archive-Sugar

6. https://www.ewg.org/research/body-burden-pollution-newborns/detailed-findings

7. Zhang, Sharon et al. "Aging and Intermittent Fasting Impact on Transcriptional Regulation and Physiological Responses of Adult Drosophila Neuronal and Muscle Tissues." *International journal of molecular sciences* vol. 19,4 1140. 10 Apr. 2018, doi:10.3390/ijms19041140

8. Fasting and release of more HGH: Ho, K Y et al. "Fasting enhances growth hormone secretion and amplifies the complex rhythms of growth hormone secretion in man." *The Journal of clinical investigation* vol. 81,4 (1988): 968-75. doi:10.1172/JCI113450

9. https://www.edisoninst.com/15-benefits-of-drinking-lemon-water-in-morning-empty-stomach/

For more connection to Dr. Sharnael and her powerFULL resources, check out her online bookstore and blog at www.swiftfire.org.

Or connect with her in her other popular classes at
www.swiftfire.org/onlineclasses

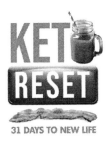

31 DAYS TO NEW LIFE

DR. SHARNAEL WOLVERTON SEHON, ND

START YOUR ONE-YEAR MEMBERSHIP NOW!

SWIFTFIRE.ORG/ONLINECLASSES discount code *"KETODISCOUNT"*

✔ Ready to start making wise healthy choices that support divine health?

✔ Ready to do this with LIKE-Minded people all with ONE focus together?

✔ Ready to RE-Member and RE-Mind the brain and body through amazing education/programming and practice?

✔ Ready to see and BE the strong Divine Health that you ARE? Ready to Re-Member and Re-Mind the tools we have to support us daily?

✔ Ready to support the body not just physically and MENTALLY but emotionally? READY TO MAKE THIS FUN AND EASY?

I am hosting a support group full of education, support, programming and FUN to RE-Member and RE-Mind our healthy sugar-free life!

There are 31 videos, articles, recipes, and LITERALLY hundreds of dollars' worth of drawings to keep you in the game. You will have access to these videos and more educational help and support with recipes, fun, tips, interactive support, high energy fellowship of like-minded folks doing this together as one.

AVAILABLE FOR PURCHASE AT:
SWIFTFIRE.ORG/ONLINECLASSES

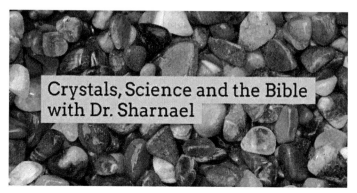

Crystals, Science and the Bible
with Dr. Sharnael

Interested in more understanding about crystals, oils and science? I have a special _Interactive_ Private Facebook Membership Class and Group!

✔ Classes and Interviews

✔ 100's educational posts

✔ How do Oils and Crystals work together?

✔ Fun high-vibe community for Truth finders

✔ Tips and Testimonies from others on the journey

✔ One-year membership to enjoy ongoing videos, classes, and educational posts

Meet others on the same path, all interacting and Re-Membering together! Joins us today!

Use Discount code "CrystalDeal4U" as my personal thank you!

Check out swiftfire.org/onlineclasses to find the Online Class section.

Interested in where I get my quality high-vibe oils? Go to my website www.drsharnael.com (member #1090401), or message me on social media @drsharnael and I will get you started!

AVAILABLE FOR PURCHASE AT:
SWIFTFIRE.ORG/CLASSES

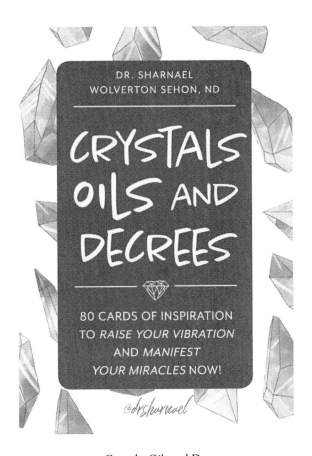

Crystals, Oils and Decrees

80 Cards of Inspiration to Raise your Vibration and
Manifest your Miracles Now!

AVAILABLE FOR PURCHASE AT:
SWIFTFIRE.ORG/STORE

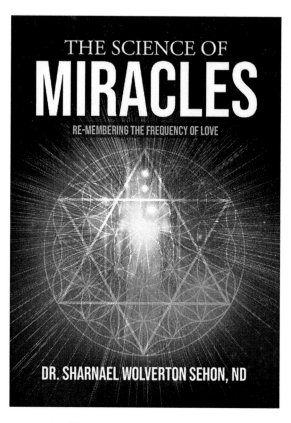

THE SCIENCE OF
MIRACLES
RE-MEMBERING THE FREQUENCY OF LOVE

DR. SHARNAEL WOLVERTON SEHON, ND

You can't pee in the pool and hope it doesn't get everywhere! With energy it is the exact same way. Issues in one area of your life affects everything. Tired of cycling the merry-go-rounds of negative patterns in your life? Join Dr. Sharnael and understand the simplified beautiful marriage of Quantum Physics and Spirit. Apply her easy formulas to your own life and experience your personal quantum leap miracles today. You deserve a Super-natural life every moment of every day. Start today!

Other popular classes and memberships By Dr. Sharnael available at
SWIFTFIRE.ORG/ONLINECLASSES

Crystals, Oils, Energy & the Bible

An interactive group of Spirit/Energy lovers on the journey together with testimonies, hundreds of educational posts, and videos.

Keto Reset 31 Days to New Life Membership

31 days of videos to reprogram you to the Keto Life. Join us for fun, accountability, testimonies, tips and recipes.

Muscle Testing

Teachings on how we can use our own bodies to know exactly what is right for us at any given time through energy (whether it's about health, oils, nutrition, crystals, relationship choices, or whatever). Includes a class and 4 demos.

I AM My Divine Partner

Exploring Conscious Choices to Re-Membering your Divine Partner NOW!

I Love My Liver/Gallbladder

Walks you through a guided 4 day Liver/Gallbladder cleanse, includes three videos and support.

Upgrades with Instagram

Simple easy steps to upgrade your IG for more followers and influence to your world.

Inspiring Your World with Video w/ Dr. Sharnael

Teaches basic steps in how to use videos for your soul purpose in business or ministry including tools, resources, simple equipment and tips to make each video look amazing.

www.swiftfire.org/onlineclasses

Personal Coaching and Consultations

www.swiftfire.org

For the Essential Oils Hook-Up, Personal coaching and consultations - Visit www.drsharnael.com (Member #1090401) or inbox me on social media and I will get you started!